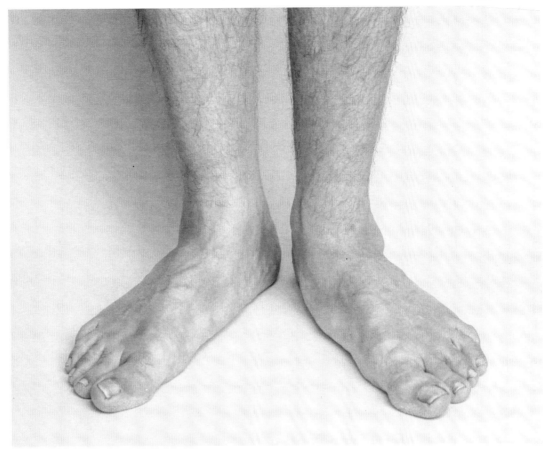

The Inverted Orthotic Technique:
A Process of Foot Stabilization for Pronated Feet

By

Richard L Blake, DPM

Past President, American Academy of Podiatric Sports Medicine
Adjunct Faculty, California School of Podiatric Medicine, Samuel Merritt
University, Oakland, California
Past Special Editor, Sports Medicine, Journal of the American Podiatric Medical
Association
38 Years Podiatrist at Sports and Orthopedic Institute, Saint Francis Memorial
Hospital, San Francisco, California

Printed in the United States of America

First Printing, 2019

The medical information contained in this book, including treatment and/or product recommendations, are solely the opinion of the author.

ISBN XXXXXXXXX

Library of Congress Control Number: XXXXXXXXXXX

Book Baby Publishing

7905 N Crescent Blvd

Pennsauken, NJ 08110

https://www.bookbaby.com/

Dedication

I would love to dedicate this book first to my wife Patty, who continues to inspire me, love me, and bring peace to my world. She is an incredible woman. We have travelled through life together for over 47 years and that has been a tremendous gift to me. I love you Patty so very much.

My second dedication is to my beloved profession. Since I decided to apply to Podiatry school in 1975, I have never looked back. Podiatry is a tremendous profession of caring for patients. This book is a reflection of this love affair with my profession and my desire to be a positive in the big picture. When I first designed an Inverted Orthotic Device for a patient many years ago, I knew that I had something special. Understanding the biomechanics of patients and how to fix them when broken or causing abnormal stress has been my life's journey. The Inverted Technique was really a natural bi-product of that journey.

And, finally, my third dedication is to my family. The demands of medicine and research can distract us from what is really important in life. My wife, my children and their spouses, and my grandchild, have all taught me to love more than I could ever imagine. It is in trying to love your family and then your patients, that the extra dedication to understanding and applying the Inverted Orthotic Device to patient care really can take hold in your practices. I believe it is worth the effort.

Forward

The practice of podiatric biomechanics was to be changed forever when Richard Blake, DPM made the decision to enroll at the California College of Podiatric Medicine in 1975. Dr. Blake was a thoughtful, energetic, and hard working student who transitioned seamlessly into the arena of fellowship training, a faculty position, and then into private practice. With his interests and dedication to sports medicine, he became aware of a situation that had perplexed countless practitioners since the specialty area of biomechanics was first developed within the field of podiatry. Why was it that orthotic devices were often unable to match the practitioner's expectations of how they should improve their patients function. One would examine their patient, obtain a cast, complete a prescription, and have an orthotic laboratory complete the device. Then, on the day of dispensing the orthotic device, there was often a feeling of surprise, as the anticipated results did not materialize. Although the patient may have experienced some improvement with the device, the outcome was often disappointing.

Personally, I experienced situations, especially in the area of podiatric pediatrics where it was not uncommon for the initial orthotic device to produce less than optimal results. This would typically lead to orthotic adjustments where additional pads, wedges and posts were applied to try and achieve the desired correction. The same situation certainly occurred in other portions of the patient population, and to a significant extent in the area of sports medicine ,where practitioners were often faced with patients who demonstrated significant abnormal function and mechanical forces.

When Dr. Blake encountered this dilemma, he developed the proverbial better mousetrap. Combining his practical knowledge of sports mechanics with functional biomechanics, he developed a device that would better support the significant abnormal dynamic forces found in athletes with abnormal lower extremity function. As he worked more and more with altering the parameters of how an orthotic device should be corrected, he developed what would ultimately be termed the Blake Inverted Orthotic Device. Initially met with some degree of skepticism due to its extreme departure from the classic Root type of orthotic device, it soon became quite clear that utilizing this technique, especially in marked overpronation, suddenly changed the playing field in successfully treating this patient population. Furthermore, it became apparent that this type of device, although originally developed for use with the athletic population, clearly would be just as effective in almost all patients demonstrating significant abnormal foot function.

Personally, it has allowed me to provide the type of control, correction, and enhanced mechanics that I have always wished for my pediatric patient population. In many instances, youngsters previously only improved with the use of a UCBL type of orthotic device or AFO, can now be treated successfully with a more comfortable and efficient device. When one looks over the landscape of podiatry and what it has provided for patients with disabling lower extremity problems, it is difficult for one to select any device that has had a more profound effect on our patient population than the Blake Inverted Orthotic Device.

Now prescribed by thousands of practitioners around the world, the philosophy of treating a patient's biomechanical problem with this type of device, along with its modifications, has certainly improved the quality of life for tens and most likely hundreds of thousands of patients. The Inverted Orthotic Device has benefited the full range of our patient population, from the athlete to the aging to the pediatric patient as well.

It has been a personal and professional honor to have known Dr. Blake from his days as a student, through his fellowship training, up to the present where we are partners in practice. I can't thank him enough for the countless hours and hard work he dedicated to developing a technique that has improved the lives of so many of our patients. This truly represents a job well done! Read the book, understand the principles, and enjoy the satisfaction of a successful biomechanics practice.

Ronald L Valmassy D.P.M.,
Past professor and Chairman
Department of Podiatric Biomechanics
California College of Podiatric Medicine

Editor
Clinical Biomechanics of the Lower
Extremity, Mosby Publishing, 1996

Inverted Orthotic Technique Pre-Test

Answers at the end of the Book on the last page

1. What is the number one function of the Inverted Orthotic Technique?
2. If a patient stands 12 degrees everted in heel valgus, what is the initial Inverted Orthotic Technique degrees ordered?
3. How does the cast correction correlate to the degrees of heel change noted for the patient?
4. What are the common muscle groups strengthened in patients who have pronation syndrome?
5. With a resting position of 2 degrees inverted, how can that be related to a pronation problem?
6. With overpronation, which knee compartment gets compressed?
7. As you attempt to eliminate or slow down overpronation, what are methods utilized to protect the lateral column from oversupination?
8. Why does equinus cause excessive pronation, in what plane primarily does it cause subluxation, and why is it important to reverse when utilizing the Inverted Orthotic Technique?
9. When designing an Inverted Orthotic Device, what landmark becomes the peak of the medial arch?
10. When performing gait evaluations, what are the 6 most common abnormal forces you are evaluating for?
11. There are 27 common areas that can get painful from overpronation listed (Appendix 1). What are the 3 most common sources of pain in the distal medial shin from overpronation?
12. Overpronation, if it is the cause or aggravating factor in an injury, affects the weakest link in the chain. If it affects a weak posterior tibial tendon, what are the 7 locations that a weak posterior tibial tendon can present with pain?
13. From simple to complex, what are the 10 methods of helping to control overpronation (for example, one of them is J strap heel inversion with leukotape and coverall to protect the skin)?
14. The Inverted Orthotic Technique is made off of what 2 casting techniques at present?
15. Why does one patient with overpronation get well with 25% pronation help and another patient needs 110% for awhile?
16. Occam's Law means that the most common cause of an injury is the cause of the injury. How does this work with the Rule of 3 in the investigation of the cause of many overuse injuries?

Table of Contents

1. Introduction to the Inverted Orthotic Technique (pages 1-5)
2. Respect for the Lateral Column with the Inverted Orthotic Technique (pages 5-6)
3. Components of Typical Inverted Orthotic Device (page 7)
4. 5 to 1 Relationship in the Inverted Orthotic Technique (pages 8-9)
5. Gait Evaluation is Crucial in the Inverted Orthotic Technique (pages 9-11)
6. Heel Bisection is Vital to the Inverted Orthotic Technique (page 12)
7. Lowering Correction in the Inverted Orthotic Technique (page 13)
8. Use in Runners of the Inverted Orthotic Technique (pages 14-15)
9. The Inverted Orthotic Technique and the Movement across the Bottom of our Feet (pages 16-17)
10. Rearfoot Varus and the Inverted Orthotic Technique (pages 17-18)
11. Lateral Column Support for the Inverted Orthotic Technique (pages 18-20)
12. Medial Column Support Enhancements for the Inverted Orthotic Technique (pages 21-22)
13. Common Indications for the Inverted Orthotic Technique (pages 23-27)
14. How Much Correction is Necessary to Help a Patient (pages 27-28)
15. 3 Approaches to Utilizing the Inverted Orthotic Technique (pages 28-29)
16. Inverted Orthotic Technique as a Process (page 30)
17. Categorizing Biomechanical Patients (page 31)
18. Initiating Treatment for the Biomechanical Patient with Over Pronation (pages 32-33)
19. When Correction Proves Too Much (pages 34-35)
20. Feel of the Foot at Push Off (pages 35-36)
21. When Correction Proves Too Little (pages 36-39)
22. Serial Orthotic Devices with the Inverted Orthotic Device (pages 39-40)
23. Growing Child and the Inverted Orthotic Technique (pages 40-41)
24. Shifting Attention from Pronation when Utilizing the Inverted Orthotic Technique (pages 41-42)
25. Varying Stress with Shoes when Utilizing the Inverted Orthotic Technique (pages 42-43)
26. What Else Helps Pronation when Utilizing the Inverted Orthotic Technique (page 43)
27. Followup Advice (pages 43-44)
28. Break In Period (page 44)
29. What Makes A Patient Stable (page 45)
30. Manufacturing the Inverted Mold (pages 45-50)
31. Conclusion (page 51)
32. Appendix 1: Pain Produced by Over Pronation (pages 52-57)
33. Appendix 2: Pain Produced by Over Supination (pages 58-64)
34. Appendix 3: 12 Point Biomechanical Outline (pages 65-67)
35. Appendix 4: Gait Evaluation and Symptoms (pages 68-84)

36. Appendix 5: Basic Components of a Lower Extremity Biomechanical Examination (pages 85-114)
37. Appendix 6: Pronation Control (Simple to Complex) (pages 115-117)
38. Appendix 7: Role and Treatment of Weak and Tight Muscles in Biomechanics (pages 117-120)
39. Appendix 8: 19 Common Foot Orthotic Cast Correction Prescription Variables (pages 121-130)
40. Appendix 9: Impression Cast Technique and Comments on Digital Scanning (pages 130-132)
41. Appendix 10: Advice for Adjustments to the Inverted Orthotic Technique (pages 133-135)
42. Appendix 11: References for the Inverted Orthotic Technique (pages 136-137)
43. Appendix 12: Answers to Self Test Questions for the Inverted Orthotic Technique (pages 138-139)
44. Index (pages 140-146)
45. Answers from Pre-Test (pages 147-149)
46. Back Cover

Introduction to the Inverted Orthotic Technique

How is the Book Structured?

It is a laboratory manufacturing process for varus rearfoot support while stabilizing the lateral column and not blocking first ray plantarflexion for propulsion. Yes, it is a mouthful. It took over 30 years to develop and test. I am proud to introduce the concept to you in these pages. I placed this video for you to review here just to have you visualize the cast correction of a high amount of inversion (3rd orthotic device for this patient). https://youtu.be/pKWOKCgJVDQ

With any new technique to your practice, it will take a lot of learning. You will have to have a good working relationship with your orthotic laboratory familiar with the various techniques discussed in the book, or at least some of them and are willing to learn. I have filled this book with study questions to help make sure that you are understanding the basic process. Where I want to expand on a concept, but not break the flow of the text, I will refer you to the Appendices near the end of the book. I promise you that this is the highest support you can offer your patients in a truly functional foot orthotic device. I divide orthotic devices into their primary function as cushioning and protective, balancing and supportive, corrective, and highly corrective. The Inverted Orthotic Technique fits into the corrective and highly corrective categories, but due to modifications or additions, you can make unlimited hybrid versions. It is truly a technique without many limits in function, except the severe supinators that will need a highly corrective anti-supination device. The technique is more part of a process of changing the biomechanics for a purpose, and this change can be varied due to different injury needs, shoe gear needs, training needs, and other variables. Basically, at times you may need full support or even temporary over correction, and other times just a little help with support and more cushion and foot protection. The book is organized around the following key areas that include:

1. Table of Contents
2. Introduction
3. Uniqueness of the Inverted Orthotic Technique
4. The Role of Gait Evaluation
5. The Role of the Biomechanical Examination
6. Categorizing Biomechanical Patients
7. Writing a Prescription for an Inverted Orthotic Device
8. Modifications to the Inverted Orthotic Device
9. How to Approach a Pronation Problem from Various Methods
10. Understanding Symptoms Related to Pronation and other Biomechanical Problems
11. Appendices for further study
12. Index

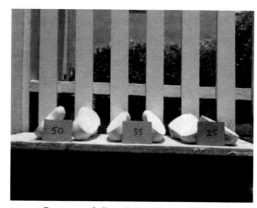

Inverted Set 25, 35, and 50

Basic Concept of the Inverted Orthotic Technique

When patients present with overpronation and have symptoms either tied to that motion or to the terrible malalignment due to their flat feet (see Appendix 1), podiatrists are left with many options. These options include various forms of foot orthotic devices, braces like the Richie Brace or Arizona Brace, shoe selections like the Motion Control Brooks Beast, strengthening exercises to fight pronation with its excessive limb internal rotation, stretching for any tight achilles or hamstrings found, gait changes for smoothness and evenness, training pattern changes for less stress and more recovery time, and then shoe modifications like midsole or outsole varus wedges and more simple power lacing. For severe pronators, all of the above categories may play some part in their overall treatment, but I want to discuss a type of orthotic device called the Inverted Orthotic Technique which I believe should be a vital aspect of your skill set.

#1 What modalities can be used to help with overpronation and its symptoms?

1. Functional foot orthotic devices
2. AFOs like Richie braces
3. Stability or motion control running shoes
4. Strengthening exercises especially for pronation control
5. Stretching of equinus forces
6. Gait changes for smoother gait
7. Training changes for less stress and more recovery
8. Shoe modifications for varus correction or overall stability
9. All of the above

(see page 138)

When a patient needs pronation support in an orthotic device, the heel position is first measured on both the right and left sides. They tend to be asymmetrical to some degree in most cases, so it is important not to just generalize. The Inverted Orthotic Technique is casted with an impression cast (Root technique) and the heel is set in the positive cast 5 degrees for every degree that you want changed (with 35 degree inversion the highest starting point). In the photo below, the resting heel position of the left foot was 7 degrees everted, and I wanted the orthotic device to center the patient's heel at vertical, so a 35 degree inverted orthotic device was ordered. The heel is measured standing barefoot (RCSP or resting position) and in the orthotic device to measure the change produced.

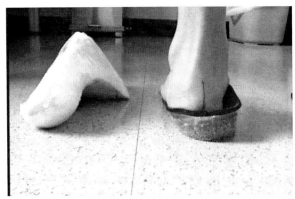

35 Degree Inverted left orthosis is being used here to correct a 7 degree everted heel at or near a vertical heel position as the goal

The Inverted Orthotic Technique, also known as the Blake Inverted Orthotic Device, or BIO, is manufactured in situations that you want a powerful inversion force at the heel and proximal arch. I invented it in the early 1980s but it took another 10 years for the technique to be field tested by my colleagues, and nurtured under the significant help by Drs Merton Root, Ronald Valmassy, and John Weed. 10 or so professional orthotic labs internationally can make the device (most with my direct initial guidance), and every laboratory can learn with some guidance. I have both a blog and YouTube channel with more information (https://drblakeshealingsole.com) about the Technique. I have just started another blog on the Inverted Technique only so that my readers can ask me questions, and the overall learning can continue (https://invertedorthotictechnique.blogspot.com).

In reality, every orthotic lab has slightly different modifications that they have found work with their clientele. Where study after study shows that modified Root devices can not significantly influence heel position (only slow the pronatory motion or intrinsically make the foot more stable), the Inverted Technique can change heel position. The Root device was initially designed to stabilize the foot in a better position and the Inverted device was designed to change foot positioning. In this way, it can exert a great effect on heel, ankle, knee and hip positions. However, with this potential of significant change, comes a greater need for the biomechanics practitioner to understand what normal and abnormal mechanics are and how they can be influenced. This information I hope will help you understand the role of the Inverted Technique in both helping normal mechanics exist and its potential to negatively impact normal mechanics. When you are used to the device created by the Inverted Technique, I hope you will see that the benefits far outweigh the negatives.

#2 Who are some of the great Podiatric minds that influenced modern day orthoses?
1. Dr. Merton Root
2. Dr. John Weed
3. Dr. Ron Valmassy
4. Dr. Kevin Kirby
5. Dr. Howard Dannenberg
6. Drs. Sheldon Langer, Justin Wernick, Joseph D'Amico
7. All of the above

(see page 138)

Where does the Inverted Technique fit into my world of orthotic devices that I prescribe for my patients? When I evaluate a patient, I try to see how I can help. As they tell me their stories, clues can present in past or present injuries, past use of orthotic devices, past selection of shoes, etc. I then watch them walk and run (if they run) and categorize their injury and gait patterns. I am sure I am not IBM Watson, but patterns can prevail. Are they pronators with pronation symptoms? Are they supinators with supination symptoms? Do they have leg length differences causing issues? Do they just have poor shock absorption problems? Has their previous treatment been perfect, or can I make some adjustments? Where do weak or tight muscles play a role? Do I start with a custom orthotic device, or do I customize an over the counter device? Of course, in the real world, patients can present with a combination of factors and your job is to figure out where to start. That is all you have to do in the first visit, and then you can slowly put things together. In terms of the pronators, is there pronation mild, moderate or severe? I did imply that the Inverted Technique can be used in anyone that you determine is a pronator with your starting point as 15 degree (mild pronator), 25 degree (moderate pronator), and 35 degree (severe pronator). Many practitioners use this starting point if they do not take measurements and are trying their best to control pronation and help their patients. I try to use the Root Balance Technique for supinators, the Hannaford for shock absorption problems, lifts for short leg syndrome, and strengthening and stretching for weak and tight muscles. I modify/customize a lot of OTC inserts, like Sole or Powerstep, for pronators also. On average, 20% of my biomechanical patients

will be getting Inverted Orthotic Devices in the near future.

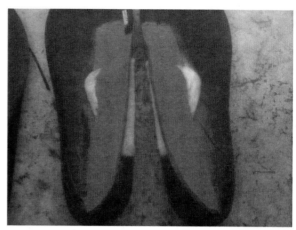

Sole OTC Inserts Customized

#3 In general, of the following causes of injuries or pain syndromes, which is the main reason that an Inverted Orthosis is prescribed?
1. Pronation
2. Supination
3. Poor Shock Absorption
4. Limb Length Discrepancy
5. Tight Muscles
6. Weak Muscles

(see page 138)

The Inverted Orthotic Technique probably stands alone for foot orthoses, except Bi- and Tri-axial devices, in the world of severe pronation, but there are many techniques for mild to moderate pronation that can also be helpful. The classic is the modified Root where you are inverting the foot over 3 degrees and then using high lateral heel cups or just stable shoes and boots (made by many laboratories). I have worked some on Dr.

Richard Lundeen's Biaxial and Triaxial techniques that also seem to get more inversion force into the foot (made through Allied OSI labs). https://www.aolabs.com/ Appendix 8 summarizes most of the orthotic devices, including those not utilizing the Inverted Technique, that I have seen on the market for more pronation correction in the modern era. My partner, the late Dr. William Olson, used KLM labs to manufacture many of these to great success. http://www.klmlabs.com/It was Dr. Olson that introduced carbon graphite devices into the profession. I am not including the classic UCBL, Roberts-Whitman plates, and Shaffer arch supports, since I have no experience with utilizing these for my patients. http://ever-flex.com/plates.html

#4 What is not a common, non Inverted Technique, device for better pronation control (from Appendix 8)?

1. Modified Root device set at 5 degrees inverted
2. Modified Root device with Medial Kirby Skive
3. Forefoot Valgus/Plantarflexed First Ray foot type poured as is
4. Forefoot Varus/Forefoot Supinatus foot type poured as is
5. Modified Root Device set at 8-10 degrees inverted with Medial Kirby

(see page 138)

Respect for the Lateral Column with the Inverted Orthotic Technique

The Inverted Technique started as a medial column force to slow down pronation and actually invert the heels of patients. My first patient had a collapsed lateral tibial plafond with increasing genu valgum and after 6 different devices I finally found that a 24 degree inversion (with hiking boots for the lateral column protection) worked. It then took 7-10 years to understand that aspect of the device, and then another 10 years to understand its effects both positive and negative on the other 3 arches. I must emphasize that I treat patients and, for all but 10 years, I have carefully made my own orthotics free to experiment and learn. I realized early in my career that I had something good to do, and I have been passionate with it. Since I treat patients, functional foot orthotic devices are a great tool to help almost every patient in any stage of injury, or for long term protection and prevention. And the type of orthotic device you use can vary during the course of an injury (from more cushion to more support for example). It was early in my development of the Inverted Technique that 3 smart practitioners helped me protect the lateral column. Dr. Mathias Fettig modified my technique for forefoot valgus/everted deformity patients to support the lateral column and I use his technique regularly. Dr. Raymond Feehery pointed out the cuboid support was crucial, and I use his modification some, and I am very careful with cuboid support in my impression

casting and mold preparation. Dr. Jane Denton showed me how I could lower the support in the office if my dispensed pair was just too inverted and creating some lateral instability. I am forever grateful to these individuals. These will be discussed further. The metatarsal arch (distal transverse arch) is a neglected arch in my mind. As podiatrists, we capture the metatarsal alignment well only in suspension casts (my impression of choice). Other techniques flatten that area too much. But, even suspension casting does not really support the bones well in some patients (only the skin outline is captured) and we are forced to use over the counter metatarsal pads on custom orthotic devices. Orthotic devices are still mired in an industry that values medial arch support over everything. 40 years ago Dr. Merton Root tried desperately to separate arch supports and functional foot orthotic devices. The Inverted Orthotic Technique, the mega medial arch support, has helped teach me the value of the lateral and metatarsal arches. The 4th arch, the proximal transverse arch, is well stabilized by the Inverted Technique and the care of the cuboid in impression casting and mold preparation.
http://www.drblakeshealingsole.com/search?q=Fettig

#5 The Inverted Technique has many modifications since its inception due to the help of many bright minds. Which of the following is not a correct match for the arch that they helped?
1. Dr. Jane Denton——-Lateral Arch
2. Dr. Kevin Kirby——-Medial and Lateral Arches
3. Dr. Mathias Fettig——-Lateral Arch
4. Dr. Raymond Feehery——-Medial Arch
5. Dr. Paul Scherer——Medial and Lateral Arches

(see page 138)

Components of Typical Inverted Orthotic Device

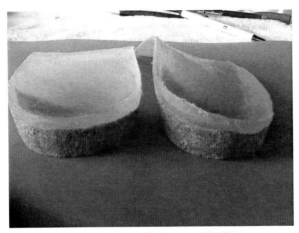

Inverted (right) Root (left)

The Inverted Device stabilizes the lower extremity by more than just the inversion. It is typically the inversion force, deep heel cups, thickness of material appropriate for the pronatory force, no motion in the rearfoot posts, and wide as the shoe. The deep heel cups are an important aspect of the famous UCBL (University of California Biomechanics Laboratory) but that is where the similarity ends. The standard Inverted Orthotic Device includes:

1. 25 degrees of inversion (5 degrees of heel change)
2. 5/32 inch or 3/16 inch polypropylene based on weight and pronation forces to be held up or slowed down
3. 23 mm heel cups both medial and lateral (deep heel cups up to 28 mm are common)
4. Zero degrees of motion in an extrinsic rearfoot post (most stable— motion used if medial knee pain or shock absorption issues)
5. Width as wide as the shoe (only if successfully allowed for first ray plantarflexion at propulsion by peaking the cast correction at the 1st cuneiform navicular joint)
6. Everything that makes the lateral column stable
7. Making sure the first metatarsal can plantarflex in propulsion

#6 If a standard 25 degree orthotic device is too rigid or stable leading to shock absorption problems, or too controlling causing lateral instability, how in the office can this be helped without making another orthotic device? I typically recommend doing one, maximum two, of these at a time and then check the patient's response.

1. Thinning of the plastic in the arch (if made of polypropylene)
2. Lowering the medial heel cup
3. Inskiving the medial heel post or removing the medial ½ of the extrinsic post
4. Grinding motion (typically 4 degrees) in the rearfoot post, but not if there is lateral instability
5. Adding a Denton Modification
6. Adding a ⅛ th inch valgus wedge (after the Denton has been tried)
7. Placing a temporary lateral Kirby between topcover and plastic heel area
8. All of the above

(see page 138)

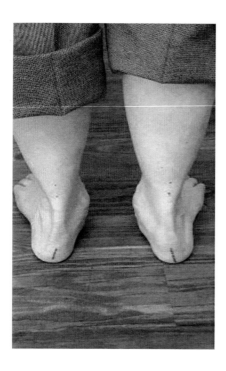

5 to 1 Relationship in the Inverted Orthotic Technique

How does the inversion work? The Inverted Orthotic Technique is a laboratory technique that is used for attempting to change heel position. After years of study, it was discovered that the current method of laboratory correction of an impression mold by 5 degrees leads to a 1 degree change in foot position. This is mainly because you only support the proximal aspect of the medial column to the navicular 1st cuneiform and then allow the plaster to gap from the foot for 1st ray plantarflexion. Therefore, 25 degrees inversion of the cast would change the foot 5 degrees and 35 degrees inversion of the cast would change the foot 7 degrees. This is substantiated daily by patients at their orthotic dispenses. You typically bisect the heel bone on the posterior surface with the patient in a prone position, then stand the patient on the ground measuring the right and left relaxed heel positions, and then re-measure with the patient standing on their orthotic devices. This should reflect the degree change of the orthotic device ordered. This standing heel position is a reflection of the middle of midstance, the most stable part of gait, before the propulsive phase begins. At times the patients respond slightly less, and at times slightly more, so this heel bisection should always be measured. This heel bisection is crucial to the technique and is based on Dr. Root's measuring technique. Some laboratories fill the arch slightly more and some slightly less and that can affect the heel change. Even standard orthotics, with or without Kirby skives, with or without medial or lateral arch modifications, or other techniques are still measured this way. Even if your heel bisection is slightly different than mine from time to time, the change in degrees should be the same. It should reflect a change in a positive direction for that patient. And, since there are so many factors which influence the change in the heel position, it is important to document the exact change so you can make plans for future corrections.

#7 Measuring the changes in heel positions by the heel bisection lines is crucial to the Inverted Technique. Which of the following influences heel positions?

1. Roundedness or Flatness of the heel as you invert the heel
2. Position of the subtalar joint axis
3. Amount of Ligamentous Laxity
4. Addition of Kirby Skive
5. Amount of Arch Fill
6. Amount of Orthotic Device lateral to subtalar joint axis
7. All of the above

(see page 138)

Gait Evaluation is Crucial for the Inverted Orthotic Technique

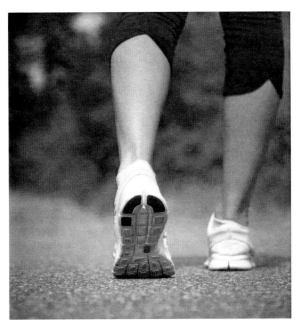

Gait Evaluation is Crucial to Analysis of Treatment

Well before you ever bisect a heel, you will have watched the patient walk with and without shoes. You will have come to some conclusion on position and motion of each foot. What are the common observations made? Start this observation barefoot. Remember that changes of 1-3 degrees are typically not seen by the human eye and you will record it as no motion.

- Inverted heel with little to no motion
- Vertical heel with little to no motion
- Everted heel with little to no motion
- Inversion motion at heel contact (typically from a vertical, inverted, or everted heel strike)
- Eversion motion at heel contact (typically from a vertical or inverted heel strike)

It is important to note that heel positioning is really only done well with the heel in the center of your eyes. Even when the foot is completely straight, the heel will be still angled anterior medial to posterior lateral. When you bisect the heel, your eyes have to be perpendicular to this angled heel with the prone patient up slightly on the examined side. Yet, that is in your control when bisecting a heel. As you watch a patient walk, you can not control the heel position, and it takes time to get good at this analysis. The further the gait is external, the further your eyes are from perpendicular to the heel, the further you are probably going to be guessing at the initial observations. If the heel looks everted, even in a highly externally rotated angle of gait, you are probably looking at a very severely valgus foot.

#8 When we watch a patient walk with and without shoes, the heel is crucial in our observations. The common observations include all but:

1. Heel everts from a vertical position
2. Heel inverts from an everted position
3. Heel everts from an everted position
4. Heel seems stationary vertical
5. Heel seems stationary inverted
6. Heel seems stationary everted
7. Heel everts from an inverted position

(see page 138)

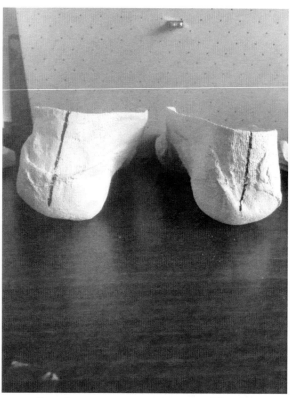

See the asymmetry captured in the impression casts of wind swept feet of over pronation left and slight varus right. This is actually what was seen in gait and the prescription should reflect this with Inverted Technique left and Root Balanced right. Remember the impression casts represent forefoot to rearfoot deformity data only, but in this case represented what I saw in gait in the rearfoot motion.

It is crucial in biomechanics to record asymmetry. For many reasons, feet tend to be different. It is normal to attempt to blend them together, but heel bisection data can keep you honest. As you watch the patient walk, try to decide what foot is more pronated or supinated. The 3 common heel observations will be:

- Vertical heel with more eversion (need to find out why the eversion)

- Everted heel with no motion (probably maximally pronated)
- Inverted or vertical heel with no motion (possibly maximally pronated)

You have made an observation of the position and motion (it gets easier the more you do). You have made an observation of the asymmetry between feet. It is now time to put their shoes on and walk first. I love when they have both new and old shoes (sometimes you have to tell them to bring some old shoes at another visit). Shoes greatly influence the patient and the prescriptions we write. A pronator barefoot can look better or worse when a shoe is placed on their feet. A supinator also can improve or decline in function. Subtle motions barefoot can be less subtle with shoes on. Pes cavus feet are some of the most interesting with over pronation in one shoe type and over supination in another shoe type (called medial and lateral instability requiring Root Balanced Technique). But, in general, the findings barefoot are highlighted with shoes. The pronation is seen more easily or the supination is seen more easily. And again, make the observation which foot looks more pronated or more supinated, since it should reflect in your prescription some way. The observations commonly made with shoes on include:

- Heel contact eversion (one side greater)
- Heel contact inversion (one side greater)
- Heel stays inverted
- Heel stays vertical
- Heel stays everted

#9 Asymmetry is a big deal in biomechanics and your treatments. Except one, what are some possible scenarios if you pay attention to asymmetry?

1. More pronation control needed in one orthotic device
2. More supination control needed in one orthotic device
3. Pronation control needed in one foot, supination control needed in the other foot
4. Lifts for a short side
5. Neutral shoe for one foot, and motion control shoe for the other foot

(see page 138)

Appendix 4: Gait Evaluation and Symptoms (pages 67-83) really explores the area of gait evaluation and how it helps with understanding the role of the Inverted Orthotic Technique.

Heel Bisection is Vital to the Inverted Orthotic Technique

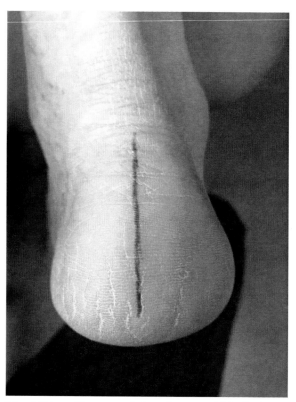

Heel Bisection crucial to Inverted Technique

Do one foot at a time. When using the Inverted Orthotic Technique, the understanding of amount of pronation observed and heel bisection data gives you ample information for your prescription.

You then lay the patient prone and bisect the back of the heel. This is discussed in the Appendix 5 but you are attempting to get the best representation of the heel you can. Then stand the patient up and look at the back of the heels. This should just make your initial observation easier with no changes. The inverted heel should still look inverted, the vertical heel still straight up and down, and the everted heel still everted. When you are learning heel bisections, this observation helps as an everted heel should not be suddenly an inverted heel due to the line you drew. Be patient with yourself. Trust the initial observation of the heel position more than your line at first. Make sure you are centering your eyes to the back of the heel.

Lowering Correction in the Inverted Orthotic Technique

It is the norm in the foot orthotic world that I see to start conservative with moderate to severe pronation or supination conditions. Because I take the opposite approach at trying to get maximal support sooner than later (although in severe cases may take me up to 3 progressive orthotic corrections to get there), I have many adjustments that I do mainly in the office. So, I need materials to get these adjustments done, and a grinding wheel to accomplish some of them. You therefore need space in the office, or second best at home, to accomplish the adjustments necessary. I trained my brother Robert to do these skills, and you can outsource some of them also.

#10 The Inverted Technique is the most scientific approach to changing heel positions, but it is still only an estimate due to many factors. Therefore, it is important to be able to lower or raise the correction several degrees each way after the orthotic device is made. This can be accomplished by which of the following?

1. Lowering the medial support (thinning the arch, narrowing the devices, lowering the medial heel cup, inskiving the medial heel post, or placing motion in the post)
2. Raising the medial support (reinforcing the arch either under the plastic or above the plastic, adding temporary Kirby medial heel area between plastic and top cover, adding ⅛ inch varus wedge, adding Morton's extension)
3. Raising the lateral support (Denton modification, ⅛ inch valgus wedge, temporary lateral Kirby, Dancer's padding, temporary Feehery cuboid support, forefoot extension under 4th and 5th metatarsal heads)
4. Lowering the lateral support (lowering lateral heel cup, lowering lateral phalange)
5. All of the above
6. Only 1 and 4 for lowering amount of varus support
7. Only 2 and 3 for raising amount of varus support

(see page 138)

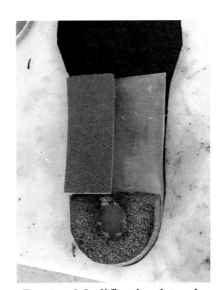

Denton Modification lateral arch right foot still needs grinding (flat to supporting surface)

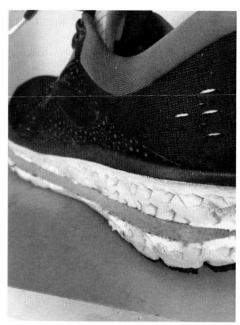

¼ inch varus midsole wedge for greater pronation control

Use in Runners of the Inverted Orthotic Technique

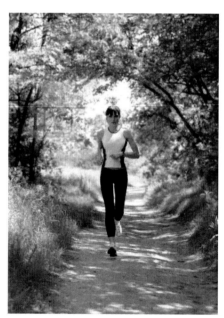

Running Gait can be totally different than Walking Gait

Let us talk about some of the peculiarities of designing running orthotic devices. With runners, you have to watch them run. The same observations as with walkers are to be made in general, but the running gait cycle is 95% pronatory with much more force than the walking gait cycle, and a little less complex. Controlling the pronatory gait cycle in runners is ideal for the Inverted Technique (capturing the runner's varus wedges I used in podiatry school). The foot strike is where you have to control the motion and it either heel, midfoot, or forefoot. An Inverted Orthotic Device will have the most effect on heel strike runners, and secondly on midfoot strike runners, although stability can be accomplished to a greater degree in midfoot strikers. If the patient is a forefoot striker, it is vital to have corrections in the forefoot extensions, and I try to get them to be more midfoot land if their motion is hard to control. It is easy to see how the running orthotic device can be totally different than the walking device at times. A pronator in walking can be a supinator in running for example, or a supinator in walking can be a severe pronator in running. The base of a standard running orthotic device can be 25 degrees inverted in 95% of all runners to start with and more forefoot control added in forefoot strikers. The observation then made in runners are:

- Foot Strike Position (heel, midfoot, forefoot)
- Heel Position at Foot Strike (inverted, vertical, everted)

- Motion Observed after foot strike (mild pronation, moderate pronation, severe pronation, or supination)

#11 The standard running orthotic device is 25 degrees inverted (a customized 5/16th inch varus wedge). Which of these general rules are not true?
1. The Inverted Orthotic Technique is great for runners with forefoot strike patterns.
2. The Inverted Orthotic Technique is great for midfoot strike patterns.
3. The Inverted Orthotic Technique is great for a supination running pattern with prolonged lateral wedge.
4. All of the above
5. 1 and 3

(see page 138)

With walking, but especially with running, shoes can make a big difference in what orthotic devices you prescribe. It can be a complex discussion, but to summarize, the amount of support needed to allow a patient to function in a relatively pain free environment is based on factors like shoe type, orthotic prescription, training stresses, running styles, etc. Therefore you can take a severe pronator, use a fairly standard orthotic device, add a motion control shoe, get their anti-pronation muscles stronger, have them train smarter and with better recovery sessions, and lessen their forefoot strike to more midfoot and you have helped them run for years. When that same patient is not motivated to get stronger or make changes in training or shoes, then they need more stability generated from the orthotic device. I have had many patients for

example in Inverted Orthotic Devices hidden within barefoot technology shoes which provide little support (as long as no one in the running community ever knows of this compromise). It is also very important when you are using powerful orthotic devices or powerful motion control shoes that pronators do not become supinators. I have had to take a lot of my pronators in stability or motion control shoes and place them in neutral shoes for that purpose. Sometimes it also becomes apparent that the shoes are almost more important than the orthotic device, and I have had to lower the orthotic support some.

#12 In general, what type of running shoe is ideal for the Inverted Technique, especially when the amount of inversion completely corrects for all of the pronation?
1. Motion Control shoes
2. Stability shoes
3. Neutral shoes
4. Minimalist shoes
5. Maximalist shoes

(see page 138)

The Inverted Orthotic Technique and the Movement across the Bottom of our Feet

It is time in our discussion to imagine the bottom of the foot when someone is walking. The patient lands somewhere on the heel influenced by all of the swing phase forces, but typically on the lateral heel, followed by contact phase pronation. Contact phase pronation with knee flexion is crucial for shock absorption and finishes the internal rotation of the entire limb. The two forces that the Inverted Technique are trying to influence is when the patient lands maximally pronated (which may be inverted, vertical or everted) and stays there (functioning a long way from an ideal stacked alignment or neutral position), or when the contact phase pronation from central or lateral heel strike is too much, too prolonged into midstance or propulsion phases, or too fast. The force you are creating with the Inverted Technique inverts the heel and rearfoot up to the navicular 1st cuneiform joint (lifting this area up) and slows down the pronatory motion. It is easy to image that this is a supinatory force on the subtalar joint. If we supinate the subtalar joint in open kinetic chain, we dramatically tighten up the range of motion of the midtarsal joint oblique axis (grab the heel, invert it and then evert it, and from each position move the oblique axis of the midtarsal joint to see how an inverted heel has tighter motion). The heel inversion places more pressure instantly on the lateral column first making the cuboid very stable (other aspects of lateral column stability are discussed below). This rearfoot inversion at the navicular 1st cuneiform allows for great peroneus longus and posterior tibial strength as they work to stabilize the midfoot. As the forefoot loads, ground reaction forces causes the midtarsal joint oblique axis to pronate locking the foot hopefully in a stable position. Here we need the weight in the center of the foot (second and third cuneiforms and metatarsals) as midstance moves into propulsion. Why? If the weight is only on the first metatarsal, there will be no first ray plantarflexion needed for propulsion, and the long axis of the midtarsal joint will become supinated and unstable. This is why Dr. Root used to have his orthotic devices very narrow at times (only to support fully the 2nd through 5th metatarsals) so as not to block first ray plantarflexion or encourage long axis supination. This is also one of the reasons Dr. Dannenberg invented the Kinetic wedge and Langer Labs had their first ray cutouts. https://www.langerbiomechanics.com/The concept of Sagittal Plane Blockaid derives from a blockage of first ray plantarflexion for normal propulsion. You did not want your orthotic device to make the foot work badly or encourage big toe joint jamming. Also, if the weight is too much on the lateral side, 4th or 5th ray problems of tailors bunions, lateral instability issues from feet to low back, and potentially propulsive phase pronatory problems as the weight needs to move lateral to medial and then to the other foot. Therefore, as the heel lifts from the ground, the weight should be on a very stable 2nd metatarsal, and the weight should be instantaneously transferred to the hallux at push off of the ground.

#13 Ideally, the weight moves through the foot from heel contact to push off from lateral heel, central midfoot, second metatarsal head and then through the hallux. In a pronatory pattern, the weight will go from lateral or central heel to medial midfoot to first metatarsal blocking first metatarsal plantarflexion. If the rearfoot does not adequately help centralize the weight, that centralization can be helped by:

1. Large metatarsal arches under 2nd and 3rd metatarsal shafts
2. First ray cutouts of the plastic
3. Narrow orthotic devices (2nd through 5th metatarsal heads)
4. Pronated orthotic devices emphasizing lateral and metatarsal arches
5. All of the above

(see page 138)

Rearfoot Varus and the Inverted Orthotic Technique

You are typically utilizing the Inverted Technique to lessen the eversion of a patient. That being said there are plenty of cases of rearfoot varus that need inversion in the prescription to invert the foot. If you treat ankle, shin, knee, and hip conditions, you will find plenty of times that more inversion force in the orthotic device is helpful like lateral meniscal issues, patellofemoral syndromes, medial shin splints, piriformis syndrome, etc. These will be discussed in Appendix 1. Of course, runners have so much more force to mitigate, that almost all runners could have the Inverted Technique. I credit Dr. Harry Hlavac, Dr. Steven Subotnick, and Dr. Richard Bogdan for teaching me about varus angled runner's wedges of ¼ to ⅜ inch. When I studied orthotic devices at Burns Podiatric Laboratory in Nebraska, I was taught 1/16 inch per degree change in an average sized patient.

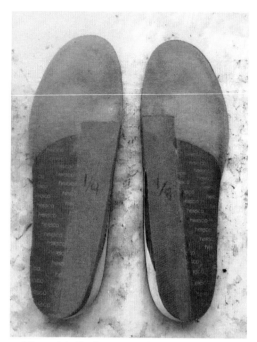

Here ⅛ (2 degrees) inch varus wedge left and ¼ inch (4 degrees) varus wedge right

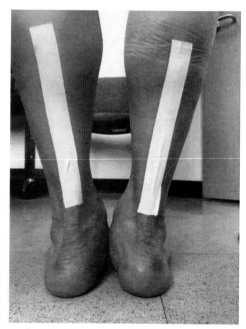

Here due to the severe tibial varum the foot is maximally pronated, and can develop pronation symptoms, even though the heels are vertical to inverted

Lateral Column Support for the Inverted Orthotic Technique

The medial arch height standards for this technique were set by 1984 and dictated by the degrees I wanted and the desire not to block first ray plantarflexion. The height of the medial arch had to stop at the navicular 1st cuneiform joint and then dropped gradually without further peaking to the anterior platform before the weight bearing surface of the first metatarsal head. I thank Root Functional Orthotic Laboratory and especially Dr. Merton Root and his widow Elaine Root, and Jeff and Kathy Root. http://www.root-lab.com/ They worked diligently with me to perfect the arch height. Most of the modifications to the technique from that point developed over the years and have been primarily to protect the lateral column and prevent the patient from becoming laterally unstable. These include:

1. Maximally pronated midtarsal joints in the impression cast to make sure the impression has a solid lateral column and fully stretched long plantar ligament. It is important that the lateral column be an exact fit under the cuboid and really the entire lateral column.

2. Most laboratories need some instruction and feedback to get the medial arch height correct. The basic tendency for laboratories when they hear about the technique is to make too high of a medial arch. This increases the chance for lateral instability and first ray plantarflexion

blockage. It must be emphasized that this is not an arch support, but a carefully organized functional foot orthotic device.

3. If there is an everted forefoot deformity, like forefoot valgus or plantarflexed first rays, you can use the Fettig modification. The Fettig modification, after Montana podiatrist Dr. Mathias Fettig, balances both the forefoot deformity laterally and the amount of inversion required by the pronation. This accounts for about 25% of my Inverted orthotic devices.

4. Lateral Column Correction is used all the time before I repress a positive cast to get more supination support. These are patients that my initial prescription overcorrected the pronation problem and I want to achieve better lateral column support. I remove any plaster expansion under the lateral column to the base of the 5th metatarsal, although not along the lateral wall. It is typically a millimeter at most.

5. The Feehery modification, after Dr. Raymond Feehery, produces a lateral column cuboid notch in the positive cast, so more plastic can support under the cuboid. I particularly use this in patients with loose midtarsal joints, especially with ligamentous laxity. Temporary Feehery modifications are used along with Denton modifications all the time.

6. The lateral Kirby, after Dr. Kevin Kirby of California, places a lateral skive from the heel contact point laterally to hold the lateral heel cup tighter. I use these for supinators, or medial-lateral instability patients, especially when the lateral heel cup is flat to the ground. I typically have to remove the lateral expansion, add the lateral Kirby, and then reapply the lateral expansion.

7. High lateral heel cups, normally the same as the medial heel cups, are 23 mm normal, and are up to 28 mm with unstable lateral ankles. Of course, shoe fit can become an issue.

8. Lateral phalanges to the plastic orthotic device run distally from the heel cup towards the front edge. This can be difficult to keep comfortable if the patient has forefoot abduction on the rearfoot, or when the foot is being held inverted. This needs the orthotic device to be as wide as the shoe so that there is no movement of the orthotic device in the shoe.

9. These lateral phalanges can just be the top cover material with soft cork or EVA reinforcement extending ½ inch superior to the orthotic device. The shoe will grab this material to make it effective, although not having it fold down while putting your shoes on can be difficult for some. All lateral phalanges are typically to the base of the 5th metatarsal and then tapered down to nothing by the distal edge of the orthosis.

10. Denton modification, after Dr. Jane Denton of California, is a simple but

powerful lateral arch fill. It runs one inch wide and from the front of the rearfoot post to the front edge of the orthotic device. It is not a valgus wedge, so should be sanded even with the supporting surface.

11. Lateral or valgus wedges of typically 1/8th inch to put a slight valgus force on the orthotic device is used in conjunction with a Denton modification. This is done in the office as a temporary fix until a new orthotic device with less inversion can be made.

12. Forefoot valgus extensions run under just the 4th and 5th metatarsal heads (typically ⅛ inch flat) or from the 1st through 5th (these are ⅛ to ¼ inch) and skived.

13. Valgus midsole wedging is typically ¼ inch and valgus outsole wedging of ⅛ inch is typical based on the shoe type or the force needed to hold the inverted position and not make the patient invert at heel contact.

Some of these modifications are demonstrated in this video on anti-supination modifications to a Root device. https://youtu.be/hMhrTmWXfDA

1. Denton Modification
2. High Lateral Heel Cup
3. Lateral Orthotic Phalange
4. Fettig Modification
5. Feehery Modification
6. All of the above
7. 1, 2, 3 only

(see page 138)

#14 Patients can be extremely pronated and yet their heel position can be close to vertical. These are patients with high degree of rearfoot varus (usually from genu varum or tibial varum "bowlegs"). Attempting to invert these patients 5-7 degrees from vertical with a 25 to 35 degree inverted device can help their pronation symptoms but can need the following lateral column accessories.

Medial Column Support Enhancements for the Inverted Orthotic Technique

The other very commonly used modifications for medial and metatarsal support are:

1. Medial Kirby Skives to the positive cast or temporary Kirbys to an existing orthotic device

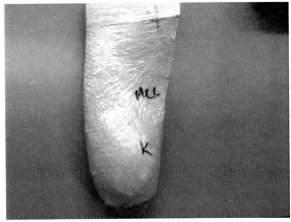

K for Kirby Skive placement
MCC for Medial Column Correction

2. Increased Medial Column Corrections (under the talus/navicular/first cuneiform) of the positive cast which is typically used with a Kirby Skive
3. Maximal metatarsal support under 2nd/3rd/4th metatarsal heads and shafts of the positive cast
4. Medial Arch Reinforcements (typically ¼ inch to 3/8 inch) to remove arch flexibility and better contact with shoe for support
5. Thicker than normal plastic (of what was previously used)
6. ⅛ inch Varus Wedge from heel to first metatarsal head (if still needed after medial arch reinforcements)
7. ¼ inch medial or varus midsole wedging or 1/8 inch varus outsole wedging
8. Metatarsal supports between plastic and top cover

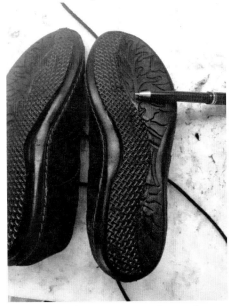

⅛ inch varus outsole wedge

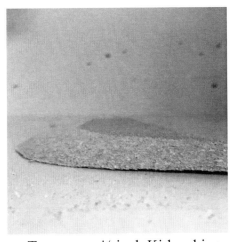

Temporary ¼ inch Kirby skive

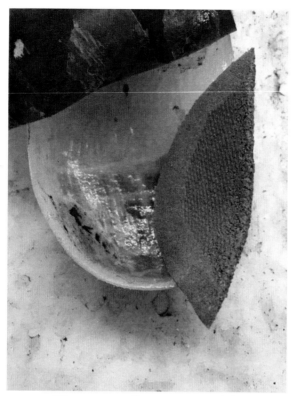

Placement of temporary Kirby skive

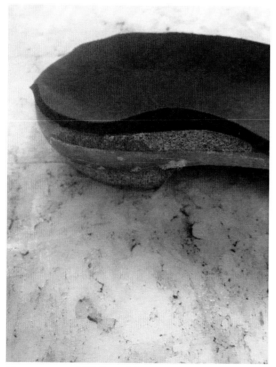

Temporary Kirby skive trimmed and in place under top cover

Common Indications for the Inverted Orthotic Technique

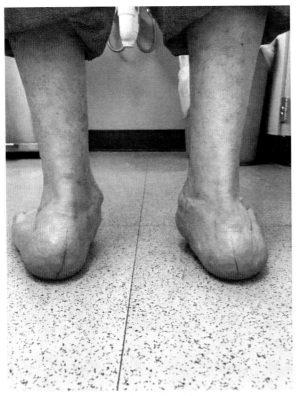

Marked Heel Valgus

What are it's present common indications for use:

1. Really Any Pronation Problem (part of this is to get the practitioner and maybe laboratory used to it then having the first one being 35 degrees)
2. Almost all running orthotics benefit from this inversion (except the 5% of runners that are supinators)
3. Moderate to Severe Pronation (this is for most practitioners)
4. Pronation from sagittal plane deformities (along with stretching equinus if appropriate)
5. Pronation from transverse plane deformities (along with strengthening external rotators if appropriate)
6. Posterior Tibial Tendon Dysfunction
7. Tarsal Tunnel Syndrome
8. Lateral Meniscal Syndromes
9. Increasing of Genu Valgum while trying to avoid knee replacement
10. Medial Shin Splints (caused by athletics)
11. Patellofemoral Syndromes (caused by athletics)
12. Juvenile or Adult Acquired Flat Feet
13. Juvenile Bunion Deformities

Let us look at this list above briefly here to get an idea of its place in the biomechanical world. The basic premise of the Inverted Technique is that it works at the control of rearfoot pronation in contact and midstance phases. The practitioner has taken an impression cast capturing the forefoot to rearfoot relationship. If this relationship is the most important aspect of the pronation syndrome (say forefoot varus or metatarsus primus elevatus), and then a Root or Modified Root device is crucial if it can support the deformity captured. This is seen commonly when 5 degrees of forefoot varus can cause a 5 degree everted resting heel position. But, if the pronation is from other sources causing contact or midstance phase pronation, then the Inverted Technique is indicated. I have also always used the Inverted Technique with high degrees of forefoot varus or supinatus since supporting those deformities with Root devices can block first ray plantarflexion at times. Try accurately supporting 12 degrees of forefoot varus and not blocking first ray plantarflexion.

#1   Really Any Pronation Problem—this is cavalier, but even mild cases of pronation can be helped with 2-3 degrees of inversion force. This would be prescribing 10-15 degrees Inverted Orthotic Devices. Of course, you can accomplish the same with Kirby Skives, or Root Devices setting the correction 2-3 inverted, but if you are new to the technique it is good to learn on smaller amounts of inversion.

#2   Almost all Running Orthoses—95% of runners land inverted and pronate 8-10 degrees before resupination. Putting a 5 degree inversion force with a 25 degree inverted orthotic device is my standard running device. It is good to see if it helps the patient's symptoms and tolerated for comfort. Of course, a 25 degree Inverted Orthotic Device functions differently in a neutral shoe, a stability shoe, and a motion control shoe. Even power lacing of an athletic shoe can make a big difference in stability.

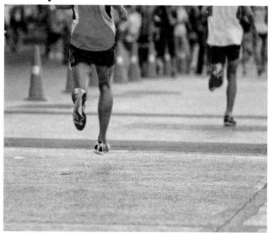

Typical Inverted Landing

#3   Moderate to Severe Pronation--typically any foot practitioner should be able to divide their patients who pronate into mild, moderate, and severe categories. The moderate and severe categories are the patients that this technique was designed for. If you are skilled in Root Biomechanics, you should be able to understand that the severe pronators are further from subtalar joint neutral than moderate pronators. But, for our discussion, let us just say that the severe pronators need a more Inverted starting point than moderate pronators. I look at orthotic devices as a process. Part of this has been influenced by the orthopedists or physical therapists I have worked with. It is totally fine to start moderate pronators at 25 degree inverted and severe pronators at 35 degrees inverted and see if it helps the patient. You progress the treatment on monthly intervals.

#4   Pronation from Sagittal Plane Deformities—A strong teaching of Dr. Merton Root was that functional foot orthotic devices worked the best with frontal plane deformities, less with sagittal plane deformities, and worst with transverse plane deformities. In a triplanar joint like the subtalar joint, when we affect one plane, we do affect the other 2 planes. However, when the force creating that triplane pronation was in a sagittal plane or transverse plane, custom foot orthotic devices had the least effect. What sagittal plane deformities cause pronation? These include tight heel cords, tight hamstrings, metatarsus primus elevatus, and leg length discrepancies.

#5   Pronation from Transverse Plane Deformities—I was paid one of the highest compliments from Dr. Root when he said that the Inverted Orthotic Technique was the best at helping pronation from transverse plane deformities. What transverse plane deformities cause pronation? These include metatarsal adductus, high vertical subtalar joint axis, internal or external tibial torsion/position, and internal or external femoral torsion or position.

#6 Posterior Tibial Tendon Dysfunction— It is not the place here to discuss the 4 stages in great detail, but Stage 4 is to be avoided and typically requires surgery. Therefore, when patients present with stages 2 and 3, I feel great pride and motivation to have them in the right orthotic device.

#7 Tarsal Tunnel Syndrome—this can be related to excessive pronation with heel eversion and a compression of the posterior tibial nerve under the laciniate ligament at the ankle. The nerve can also be compressed by inflammation in the anti-pronation tendons (PT, FHL, and FDL) that run under the laciniate ligament. It can be partially a Double Crush problem, where pronation slightly irritates the nerve at the foot and ankle, but the main issue is sciatic nerve compression above the foot (behind knee, within the hamstrings, piriformis, or low back).

#8 Lateral Meniscal Problems—typically varus correction of the heel, opens up the lateral joint line and decompresses the stress on the lateral knee compartment or lateral meniscus. It can be tricky, as you sometimes have to over correct the foot to help the knee, so watch for signs and symptoms of excessive supination.

#9 Increasing Genu Valgum—This is how the Inverted Technique started with compression of the lateral compartment and medial collapse of the knee. It can be a temporary device while the patient waits for a knee replacement, or worn for a longer period indefinitely.

#10 Medial Shin Splints—In 1984 I first presented the Inverted Technique to the Root Laboratory Seminar. In 1985, at the next meeting, Dr. Ross Leonard from Oregon presented to the group that he had gone back and remade orthotic devices on 19 of his patients that the original orthotics had not helped their shin splints. He reported success at resolution of the medial shin splints in 18 of these 19 patients.

#11 Patellofemoral Syndrome—When I first started at Saint Francis Memorial Hospital in San Francisco, I was the only podiatrist in an orthopedic clinic. Most of my patients had knee problems, like patellofemoral syndrome. The problem was a transverse plane issue of the femur coming medially too far, and the tight vastus lateralis subluxing the patella laterally. The power of the Inverted Orthotic Device needed to stop medial motion of the femur by placing a laterally pushing force on the medial side of the heel. I had to push the device as far as possible in inverting the heel without causing lateral instability. These were my first group of patients that I learned to protect the lateral column.

#12 Juvenile or Acquired Flat Feet—By 8-9 years old, Dr. Ronald Valmassy of the California School of Podiatric Medicine said that children should outgrow any heel valgus they previously had. So, 8-9 years old has become the age when deciding on surgery or orthotic devices. Parents of these children who have been managed in OTC prefab orthotic devices are shocked to learn their child at 9 now needs flat feet surgery. Children outgrow orthotic devices quickly (about every 2 shoe sizes) and need replacements. However, a growing child's foot is precious, and I would not trust its development in a prefab. The goal should be a vertical heel unless high rearfoot varus dictates the heel to be in 2-3 degrees of varus positioning. By measuring the heel position with and without orthotic devices, and all through the growth of the child, you have endeared these parents to you forever. I make custom Inverted Orthotic Devices in patients as young as 2 (actually my son Christopher started at 18 months when my wife complained she had to carry him too much for a healthy child).

Adult Acquired Flat Feet from Posterior Tibial Tendon Dysfunction or collapse from equinus forces or gradual breakdown from injury or ligamentous laxity, etc, can tolerate high corrections even at 75 years old or older. Some of my senior patients for some reason or another are not surgical candidates, at least in their minds. My job is literally to keep them moving and they can be totally surprised and overjoyed at how well they are doing. One of my best examples recently is Steven. Steven presented 14 everted right side and 18 everted left side with collapsed midfoot and 25-30 degrees angle of gait. His shoes were severely broken down and everted at initial presentation adding to the problem. At present, his heel positions in the orthotics

alone are vertical right 5 degrees everted left. Who would not say that looks good?

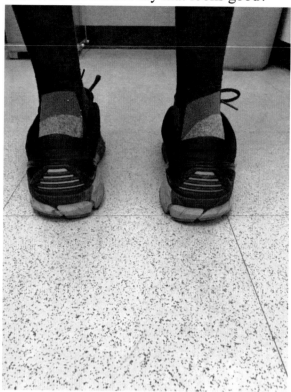

Inside of these Motion Control Brooks Beast Running Shoes are 45 Degrees Orthotic Devices with Kirby and Medial Column Corrections (the patient is functioning fairly perfectly)

#13 Juvenile Bunion Deformities—When children present with surgical bunions at 10-20 years old, knowing the life expectancy of bunion surgery without fusions (first MPJ or Lapidus), I approach it two ways: surgery followed by conservative treatments to improve the joint function, or just conservative treatment to improve the joint function. I have to design an orthotic device that centers them, demonstrates no functional hallux limitus, typically has a dancer's pad to float the first metatarsal head. This may be with any type of orthotic devices, since it is based on individual biomechanics and the goal is to eliminate functional hallux limitus. Yoga Toes, toe separators, and Correct Toes are also part of their programs. Physical therapy is used to learn abductor hallucis strengthening and mobilization of various soft tissues like to release the lateral capsule of the big toe joint. One way that you insure the bunion will get worse is design an orthotic device that they still pronate into, causing a dorsal jamming of the first metatarsal. The Inverted Orthotic Device can be a big help.

#15 Medial Shin Splints can be caused by which 2 powerful muscles which act to decelerate pronation at heel contact?
1. Posterior Tibial
2. Gastrocnemius
3. Soleus
4. Semitendinosus
5. Flexor Digitorum Longus
6. 1 and 2
7. 1 and 3
8. 2 and 5

(see page 138)

How Much Correction is Necessary to Help A Patient

The concept of how much correction to design into an orthotic device is important here. If we are talking about changing biomechanics to help injuries (the bulk of my practice), slight changes to pronation (20% correction) can be enough at times. But, I am asked daily by my patients to perfect their biomechanics (85% to 100% correction) in order to allow their injuries to heal or to indefinitely prevent surgery or relapses. I need to know how to be perfect at times, and when less than perfect at times is okay. Some patients come into the office with mild pronation and an injury caused or aggravated by pronation. Here my perfecting their biomechanics may be 2-3 degrees of varus support. Other patients present with knee pain or tarsal tunnel or posterior tibial related to their severe pronation, and only corrections up to 15 degrees will help. This has brought me great satisfaction that I can help these patients avoid a knee replacement, not allow chronic nerve pain to become CRPS, or not allowing their posterior tibial tendon to fail and progress to flatfoot surgery. Dr. Merton Root was very observant when he said that perfect orthotic therapy will fail with tight or weak muscles. This holds especially true with ligament lax patients. You can make the ideal orthotic device for a pronator with posterior tibial tendonitis, but the treatment will fail if you do not make their weak posterior tibial tendon strong, their -10 degrees dorsiflexion normal, and have them lose 40 lbs if they need to.

#16 The concept of "How Much Correction is Needed" clearly states the following:
1. 2-3 degrees of pronation control is always needed
2. 100% of pronation control is needed to help injuries caused by pronation
3. Different corrections are needed for different scenarios
4. Corrections for pronation do not always help injuries
5. 2 and 3
6. 3 and 4

(see page 138)

3 Approaches to Utilization of the Inverted Orthotic Technique

There are three approaches that podiatrists start with the Inverted Orthotic Technique: 1) for any abnormal pronation, 2) by the degree of pronation noted in gait evaluation that they can not control with their standard approaches, or 3) by the exact degree of heel inversion desired typically decided by their biomechanical measurements. Let us look at all three approaches.

You can use the Inverted Orthotic Technique for any pronation problem. Typically 10 degrees of the Inverted Technique will give you a 2 degree inversion force and is the lowest amount prescribed. This amount of correction can be achieved with standard techniques (like Root Balanced to Vertical then a Medial Kirby Skive or simply putting 2 degrees of inversion in the initial correction), but some prefer to use the inverted technique even for smaller amounts of change desired.

You can use the Inverted Orthotic Technique as Plan B in your quest to stabilize a patient with significant pronation. It takes awhile with this technique to learn how much correction to order when you are not really quantifying it, but it can be accomplished. If you use your standard technique, but the pronation continues to cause symptoms, you can use 15 degrees inversion for slight correction, 25 degrees inversion for moderate correction, and 35 degrees for significant correction in your next prescription order. Remember, for any patient, finding the right amount of stability that will give you symptom relief can be a challenge. It seems some problems need 20-30% pronation control, whereas others may need 110% (especially as we aim the correction up the chain to help shin, knee, and hip issues).

I prefer to use the biomechanics I was taught, measure the relaxed calcaneal stance position (also called resting heel position), remembering to separately correct the right and left sides, and order the inversion based on this. So, if I measure 5 degrees everted right heel, and 3 degrees everted left heel, I would then order a 25 degree inverted device for the right side, and a 15 degree inverted device for the less pronated left side. I will not dispense more than 35 degrees initially, since it makes a lot of change, and the body can struggle getting use to it. And remember the higher the inversion, the more attention you have to place on a stable lateral column. Stabilizing the lateral column typically involves an impression cast maximally pronated in the midtarsal joint to get a stable long plantar ligament and cuboid, the lateral heel cups and lateral phalange get higher as the correction gets higher (23 mm with 25 degrees and 25 mm with 35 degrees), Fettig Modification when there is a high forefoot valgus deformity yet moderate to severe pronation, no motion in the rearfoot post (since the motion comes from de-stabilizing the lateral column), Feehery modification with unstable midtarsal joint like ligamentous laxity, and utilizing a Denton Modification is common.

#17 When using the Inverted Orthotic Technique, many doctors prefer to use it for all their pronation problems. Which of the following is not a reason for that approach?

1. It familiarizes the provider with the approach on a routine basis
2. The doctor uses it for both simple and complex cases of pronation which helps with the learning curve
3. It is helpful for every foot type and pronation issue
4. If unfamiliar with the process, the doctor will understand instantly that there are other methods of helping the patient with pronation

(see page 138)

The Inverted Orthotic Technique as a Process

I work with both physical therapists and orthopedic surgeons on a daily basis. They practice a process of getting a patient better. When something does not work, they move on and experiment with a different treatment approach. The Inverted Technique is more like a process. I like to tell my patients who need orthotic devices, that it is a process, and that there is no perfect orthotic for them. It depends on the shoes they wear, the amount of correction needed now to help their problem, how strong they are, how stable their gait, and so on. The reason I mention this is that it involves the patient in the process. They intuitively understand they may need different orthotic devices for walking versus running, athletic shoes versus dress shoes, after a knee replacement that changed their mechanics, when protecting a broken sesamoid, or recovering from a knee injury. I try to impress on them that orthotic devices are a means to an end and can be manipulated to help us with more or less support at times.

#18 Orthotic therapy is a very fluid process, and should be considered a process. Which of the following statements is false?
1. There is an ideal orthotic device for each patient that you should strive for
2. If I make the best orthotic device for the patient there should never be adjustments needed
3. Since all injuries have mechanical roots, a stable orthotic device should help all injuries
4. The manufacturing of soft based orthotic devices which do not support the intrinsic foot structure ideally should never to used.
5. All of the above
(see page 138)

I have been extremely blessed by this invention, and have spent my life studying every facet of it. I have also been cursed by it since it defines who I am in my beloved profession, and I think I am so much more. It is in this psychological realm that I need to write this book. Personally, I use Inverted Technique for all pronators (yes, everyone), the Root Balance Technique for all supinators, the Hannafords for all shock absorption problems, and limb length difference treatments for patients with hip and back issues and many asymmetrical athletes.

#19 Match the correct type of orthotic device with the following abnormal functions (short leg syndrome, supination, shock absorption issues, and pronation).
1. Inverted Orthotic Technique
2. Root Balance Technique
3. Hannaford Technique
4. Heel or Full Length Lifts
(see page 138)

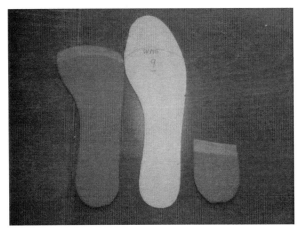

Most Full Length Lifts are cut off at the toes

Categorizing Biomechanical Patients

When I take on a biomechanical patient, I first want to categorize them as pronators, supinators, limb length discrepancy patients, shock absorption or cushion patients, weak muscle patients, or tight muscle patients. I am looking for what to treat first to give me the best results. And what does it mean to be a biomechanical patient? These are patients that my focus is off the acute injury, and into the causes of the injury in the first place. These are patients that present with overuse injuries or pain syndromes that may have some biomechanical cause or aggravating factor. There is the Rule of 3 with overuse injuries. Rule of 3 with overuse injuries. Rule of 3 means that there may be 3 causes of any injury and if found and corrected you can lessen the chance of reinjury and speed up overall healing. And, in reality, these biomechanical patients can come in with a slew of issues to sort out and help them with. It can just take awhile. So, my severe pronator, may also have tight Achilles, weak soleus and glutes, a short leg, and poor shock absorption from his shoes.

#20 Which one of the following is not a common compensation problem caused by tight achilles tendons?
1. Achilles tendonitis
2. Pronation problems due to midfoot breakdown
3. Anterior or posterior knee pain due to genu varum forces
4. Metatarsal problems due to excessive downward forces on the metatarsals

(see page 138)

Initiating Treatment for the Biomechanical Patient with Over Pronation

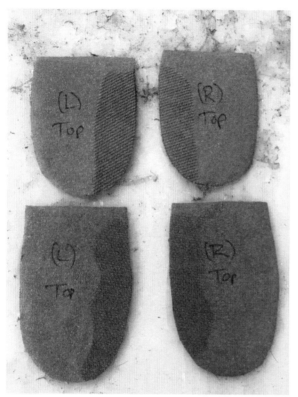

2 different lengths of ¼ inch varus heel wedges for pronation control

It is the first visit with the patient and I have determined that their problem may be helped by the correction of the pronation that I see. Typically, in my clinic, I need to have them schedule an hour visit for orthotic evaluation and casting. I love to start however on that first visit with over the counter arch supports (Sole or Powerstep are my go to types) for medial column support, or ¼ to ⅜ inch varus heel wedges if I am looking for more ankle or above the ankle improvement. It is easy to stock these, or pre cut these, in various sizes ahead of time. Sometimes, at the first or second visit, I can customize the arch support based on their gait function for even better support. Based on their problem related to the over pronation, I will teach them some form of taping to help, and get them doing a home program of some exercises. With all pronators, I love to find out why they pronate. My gait evaluation has categorized them mild, moderate, and severe. But what is actually the cause or causes of this pronation problem? This is where some version of a biomechanical examination is crucial. It can be easy to go through the following checklist of causes of overpronation. This includes:

- Frontal plane abnormalities of genu varum, genu valgum, tibial varum, tibial valgum, or forefoot varus
- Sagittal plane abnormalities of short leg syndrome with limb dominance, tight hamstrings, tight achilles, and metatarsus primus elevatus
- Transverse plane abnormalities of internal or external femoral rotation, internal or external tibial rotation, high subtalar joint axis, and metatarsus adductus
- Weak muscles include weak external hip rotators, weak gastrocnemius or soleus, weak posterior or anterior tibial tendons, weak peroneus longus, and weak intrinsic muscles

With pronators, I am looking for pronation causes at each visit until I am happy I have them all. It is the second visit in moderate to severe pronators that I am completing my biomechanical evaluation. There is an

33

overlap in the moderate group, since the mild to moderate pronators may continue with over the counter inserts, customized with varus wedging, if they are feeling great progress. Some seem to go to custom orthotic devices, others do not. There are so many factors.

#21 What are the common causes of pronation that I can evaluate in an office setting?

1. Weak Posterior Tibial or Anterior Tibial Tendons
2. Weak Peroneus Longus Tendon
3. Weak Gastroc-Soleus Complex
4. Weak Foot Intrinsic Muscles
5. Tight Achilles Tendons
6. Tight Medial Hamstrings
7. Tight Iliopsoas Tendon
8. Excessive External Angle of Gait
9. Genu Valgum
10. Tibial Valgum
11. Tibial Varum
12. Forefoot Inverted Deformities
13. Metatarsus Primus Elevatus
14. Ligamentous Laxity
15. All of the above

(see page 138)

Let us now discuss patients and common issues that come up daily in my practice concerning the Inverted Orthotic Technique. These include:

- Correction proves too much
- Feel of the foot at push off
- Correction proves too little
- Discussing with the patient the concept of "Serial Orthoses"
- Discussing with the parent of a growing child
- Discussing shifting attention away from pronation control
- Discussing shoe changes and shoe alternating
- Discussion of what will help their bad flat feet
- Discussion of follow up
- Discussion of break in period
- Discussion of what makes a patient biomechanically stable

When Correction Proves Too Much

Correction proves too much for the patient can occur in 3 ways. First of all, the patient walks and/or runs in their new orthotic devices and feel like they are moving laterally. You may or may not observe this lateral slide, but it is a strong sensation for the patient, and a sensation of instability. You ask them to tell you where they are rolling off their feet, across which metatarsals, and they say the lateral metatarsals (3,4, and/or 5) if the roll keeps them lateral weight bearing throughout midstance. Normal roll is a sense of evenness with all the metatarsals, or some sense that the 2nd metatarsal is involved (1 and 2 or 2 and 3). It is the metatarsal roll, not the hallux pushoff you want to know about. Patients can get confused about this. Secondly, the patient is wearing too controlling shoes (motion control or stability even), or too broken down shoes with a lateral heel varus bias. In both of these environments, you should not adjust the orthotic device (actually do not make any judgement on the overall control or correction), until they come back with better shoes. I never tell them to buy new shoes until they get their new orthotic devices because they may take a half size bigger, so their corrective shoes may have been what they used to need. If the shoes are old, a new shoe may be all they need. Thirdly, if the correction is too much, they may complain of supination symptoms (see Appendix 2). Commonly, it is medial knee pain from medial knee overload, or peroneal strain from overworking the lateral ankle stability muscles, or iliotibial band symptoms from the IT band overworking to protect the lateral sides of the knee and hip, or sacroiliac symptoms from jamming superiorly. You protect the patient at dispense by telling them to never push through pain, and blame any new ache or pain on the new orthotic devices. I tell them that it is okay to only be wearing them a short time, since it is good to be cautious. 30% of my patients will need an adjustment or two until the correction allows them to wear them all day and most activities.

Once you take care of any shoe issues or believe that the shoes have no bearing on the over correction, the following can be done to any orthotic device that is throwing the patient lateral (if the patient can feel it, or I can see it, then I prefer to do one thing at a time in the office visit setting until the problem is solved which could take several visits):

1. Add Denton Modification to stabilize the lateral column immediately, and with any orthotic device
2. Inskive the medial aspect of the rearfoot post
3. Grind 4 degrees of motion into the rearfoot post if they are complaining of medial knee or other supination symptoms, but not if they are already feeling unstable
4. Add a temporary lateral Kirby skive between the plastic and top cover in the lateral heel cup area
5. Lower the medial heel cup about 3 mm and narrow the width of the orthotic medial arch distally about 3 mm

6. Remove the medial ½ of the rear foot post

7. Thin the medial arch plastic based on where the patient feel the pressure the most (near the heel, height of the arch, or near the front).

This is the exact order I prefer to do this type of adjustment.

#22 The patient presents with definite overcorrection symptoms, what is not a remedy?
1. Flat post the orthotic device
2. Add Denton
3. Add temporary lateral Kirby
4. Thin the medial width
5. 2 and 3

(see page 138)

Feel of the Foot at Push Off

Feel of the foot at push off has become an essential part of my discussion of stability with patients and their education when buying shoes. When they have over pronation, they need to purchase shoes that help their weight bearing not just through the first metatarsal and big toe, but on to the second metatarsal and 2nd toe some. Patients do get good at this feel. Especially, if they have 3-4 pairs of shoes to compare, they can choose the best functioning ones. I do not want the push off to be all first, or 4th and 5th. I want more centered weight bearing, typically involving the second metatarsal and second toe. At orthotic dispense, I make my observations silently, grading myself for the performance of orthotic devices, but then I want them to focus one foot at a time, and analyze where the weight is going through the front of their foot (1st only, some involvement of 2 or an even distribution, or more 3, 4, and 5). Again, as just mentioned, this is the sense of the metatarsals and not the toes since they should push off the big toe. Things happen internally inside of the shoe that I can not see, but in general my observations should match the patient. With the inverted orthotic device, you are actually doing 2 different functions at times. Mainly, you are inverting the foot from everted to vertical (therefore the discussion above should apply). But, at times with rearfoot varus, you are inverting the foot from vertical to inverted, so you want the weight to be more lateral, but never only on the 4th and 5th metatarsals.

#23 In what instance, after designing a proper orthotic device, do you want the patient to feel that they are pushing off through the lateral half of their foot at times?

1. Forefoot Varus Correction
2. Forefoot Valgus Correction
3. Rearfoot Varus Correction
4. Rearfoot Valgus Correction
5. External Tibial Torsion Correction

(see page 138)

When Correction Proves Too Little

Correction can prove to be too little will occur in many ways. First of all, the foot change from the orthotic devices dispensed was not the standard 5:1 ratio, but more like 8:1 or so. This is actually more the cast correction ratio for children's pronated feet that Dr. Ronald Valmassy teaches in podopediatrics. I am usually disappointed (even though I know it can happen), and I make sure that the patient knows. I will check the molds and make sure the medial arch or medial heel was not lowered too much and I just did not catch it (I check every mold before pressed for issues like this). I typically grade my orthotic corrections A, B, C, etc or 100%, 90%, 80%, etc. Normally, I try to estimate what I need to take the correction to 100% or A grade and document that expected correction. If the patient's need of correction is for 100%, for example flat foot and stage 3 PTTD attempting to avoid surgery, or sesamoid fracture trying to avoid surgical removal, I just go ahead and redo the one or both orthotic devices. If the patient's need of correction is unknown, for example we are reducing pronation for chondromalacia patella symptoms, or plantar fasciitis symptoms, we may see how the next 2 months goes with their rehabilitation and symptoms before any permanent redo. Basically, we will have the patient prove that they need more support by a slower course of progress. But, I will still grade the orthotic devices and let the patient know that the correction could be improved if symptoms persist. Secondly, the correction was being staged in the first place. A recent example of a patient I have used with 14 degrees everted right heel and 18 degrees everted left heel presented with adult acquired flat foot. With my standard starting point 35 degrees inverted, or a 7 degree heel change, I predicted 3 pairs of orthotics 3-4 months apart to bring the feet to heel vertical (which he had the range of motion to do so on examination). In highly everted patients like these, I typically stage the orthotic devices to get the heel to vertical like this:

1. 35 degree inverted, 25 mm heel cups, zero motion rear foot post, width as wide as shoe, 5/32 inch polypropylene, Motion Control Shoes, and power lacing (the orthosis alone is up to 7 degree correction, and up to 2 degrees with the motion control shoe with power lacing). This may be up to 9 degrees of correction.

2. At repress of the original cast, I add a Medial Kirby skive, medial column correction only to the navicular 1st cuneiform joint, and upping to 3/16 inch polypropylene, usually gives 3-4 more inversion degrees, without changing the initial 35 degree inverted orthotic device. Now our proposed correction is 12-13 degrees of inversion force. In my patient above, the right foot was at heel vertical and the left still 5 degrees everted.

3. The initial 35 degree inverted orthotic device is reset to 45 degrees without removing the initial platform. A remedial medial Kirby is crucial to get the plantar heel surface flat from the lateral contact point and

a smooth transition into the proximal arch. This can be also improved with medial arch reinforcement and ⅛ inch varus wedge from heel to 1st metatarsal head. I am normally now still using 3/16 inch polypropylene with 28 mm heel cups. With these changes, up to 5 more degrees of pronation control can be achieved. In my patient, these changes were done only to the left side to basically get both feet functioning straight.

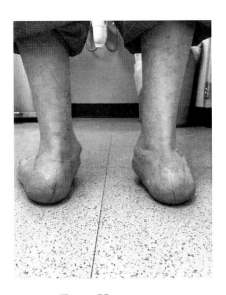

From Here

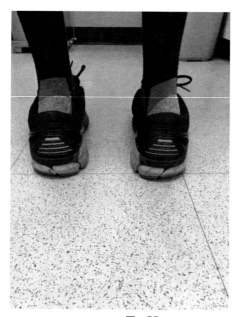

To Here

I have found over the years of going to high corrections over 35, and definitely over 45, that I am actually losing the original foot shape too much, and my correction. Therefore, the above strategy is my current recommendation. Thirdly, the correction is too little, at times when we are dealing with a problem above the foot. This can occur with knee, and sometimes hip, problems, when to help center the knee you have to overcorrect the foot. The easiest example is taking a normal foot with genu valgum and patellofemoral symptoms. At times, you need to take that normal foot and make them inverted by 5 degrees. The difference between a stable over-correction and unstable lateral instability is not the inverted position, but how well you can stabilize the lateral column with all the tips mentioned above. When you are in an over-corrected position, and it is the same as being put in a cast, the goal is to normalize the situation as soon as possible. In the scenario I just gave you, the over-correction may be necessary

for 3-6 months as you work on anti-inflammatory measures, knee bracing or taping, gait changes, physical therapy, strengthening and flexibility work, and cross training. But, even when your patient is feeling great, if the patient is in an over-correction, you must gradually normalize the mechanics. What is overcorrection in this case? Overcorrection is inverted from neutral, not just inverting the foot back to or close to neutral as we normally do.

When a patient comes into the office with an under corrected orthotic device, and you think that their symptoms would get better if you improved their biomechanics, during one or two office visits you can improve the situation by:

1. Adding a ¼ inch medial arch reinforcement
2. Adding a ⅛ to ¼ inch temporary medial Kirby
3. Adding a ⅛ inch varus wedge heel to first metatarsal head

#24 Which of the following is not a typical reason for undercorrection of the overall foot pronation?

1. You expected needing 2-3 orthotic devices with increasing pronation control right from the first visit
2. The equinus forces are too great for the control you gave
3. The weak posterior tibial or soleus muscles continue to allow the foot to pronate excessively

4. Correcting the foot mechanics perfectly does not do enough for knee positioning
5. Due to ligamentous laxity, or shoe type selection, the functional orthotic device made was subpar in correcting the foot enough to help complete correction
6. All of the above

(see page 138)

Serial Orthotic Devices with the Inverted Orthotic Technique

Discussing with the patient the concept of "Serial Orthoses" is reserved for patients at the extremes of mechanics (severe pronation or severe supination) or when the type of orthotic device to help their symptoms may still be a mystery. The severe pronation aspect is simplified if you use heel bisection data as my example earlier with the resting heel everted position 14 degrees on the right and 18 degrees on the left. Since I will only start with a 35 degree correction (7 degrees on average heel change), and then allow them to break into the device, get normalized to it for several months, before I will attempt increases, the concept of needing more than one orthotic device seems elementary. But, so many patients with pain issues just can not tolerate, or not helped, with your first attempt. They may even bring in a box of previous orthotic devices that have not worked for one reason or another. No matter what I make for the patient, or what type of adjustments I have to make, I try to understand the whys of each adjustment, so I can make a hybrid orthotic device of some sort. If they have previous orthotic devices, finding out the whys of their intolerance problem will be crucial going forward. I am though frustrated at how many patients just do not know that answer. I am always dealing with 3 arches that need more or less support. I am always dealing with the amount of material flexibility, or rigidity, or cushion required. Tarsal Tunnel Syndrome is a great example of how you can do the most perfect support ever, but if the nerves in the arch are too sensitive, the arch will have to be adjusted down, sometimes even to non-existence and getting support with Medial Kirby Skives and no medial arch to get pronation control. The more you discuss this at the start of your treatment, the more that the patient will understand and be comfortable with this approach.

#25 Making serial corrections for a complicated patient is common in a biomechanics practice for the following reasons except:
1. Extreme amounts of pronation
2. Extreme amounts of supination
3. Previous problems with orthotic devices
4. Having many different styles of shoes
5. All of the above

(see page 138)

Growing Child and the Inverted Orthotic Technique

Discussing with the parent of a growing child is a financial issue most of all that the child will need new orthotic devices every 1 and ½ to 2 shoe size changes. This can be a big issue until they have stopped growing their feet (girls 12-14 and boys 14-16). I want the children to wear their orthotic devices until they are 22 over 80% of the time of activity. This is when the adult foot really becomes tight and stable. It is when they lose their "baby fat". As they grow, and their foot is in normal foot/ankle/leg alignment by way of the orthotic device made, they have a chance to have strong stable feet with normal alignment. This has been documented to work with 20 degrees inverted orthotic devices in the articles listed in Appendix 11. I would not trust this wonderful precise development on prefabricated over the counter inserts. I would only trust my ability to make a custom orthotic device that keeps them centered at heel vertical and does not jam up the first ray or some other abnormal force. I know with my Root theory biomechanics that I can design a stable orthotic device that "does no harm" to these growing children.

#26 Which is not a general rule for designing orthotic devices for children?
1. Prefabricated devices are just as effective as custom devices until 9 years old

2. Orthotic devices for children must be remade every 1 and ½ to 2 shoe size changes
3. Boys tend to stop growing (especially at the feet) after girls
4. At 22 years old, the orthotic devices typically can no longer change arch structure, only stabilize mechanics

(see page 138)

Shifting Attention from Pronation with the Inverted Orthotic Technique

Discussing shifting attention away from pronation control when that aspect is under control but there are other factors that need to be addressed takes a lot of effort. Both my patients and I typically need to focus on one aspect at a time. So I spend the first 3-4 visits getting the right correction of orthotic device for their problems. Normally the patients are happy, they have the orthotic devices that they came in for initially, or at least I used in my treatment plan. The control of pronation may be the most important part of the treatment, or just a part that can help in the overall scheme of the patient's health. In each of these initial visits, examination and historical review continues, while the mechanics, the amount of inflammation, and the amount of neuropathic pain is assessed and treated. You may be dealing with getting them through the Phases of Rehabilitation: Immobilization, Re-Strengthening, and Return to Activity. So, as I deal with the mechanics of pronation, the inflammation and nerve pain has to be addressed. I try to determine if there are other mechanical factors at play: shock absorption issues, leg length discrepancy, tight muscles, and weak muscles. These factors can require prescriptions to physical therapy, shoe changes, or just home exercise programs.

#27 When treating patients, what is the treatment biomechanically that should be first?

1. Pronation Control
2. Short Leg Syndrome with Lift Therapy
3. Weak Muscles with strengthening exercises
4. Tight Muscles with equinus stretching
5. Depends on what is deemed the most important for each patient

(see page 138)

Varying Stresses with Shoes when Utilizing the Inverted Orthotic Technique

Discussing shoe changes and shoe alternating is a way to vary the stresses day to day or 3-4 hours at a time to help in the rehabilitation of the patient. Therefore, I do not mind if my patients alternate between orthotics of different corrections or between neutral, stability, or motion control shoes at times. I rarely mind my runners alternating between barefoot, traditional, and maximalistic shoe types if my evaluation can not see anything harmful. I want them to find any patterns of pain, like one orthotic device and one type of shoe being the most painful. This would be the combination to avoid. But, changing the stresses is great for overall healing and a great rehabilitation technique of strengthening. I think it is important to find the ideal support (95-100% support) as your gold standard, but I do not want the patient stuck in that rigid world the rest of their life.

#28 The concept of cross training works with varying shoes or orthotic devices also in injury rehabilitation and training techniques. What are the common types of running shoes that will affect biomechanics and injuries that can be varied at times?
1. Maximal Stability
2. Maximal Cushion
3. Neutral
4. Supination Control
5. Minimal Shoes
6. 1, 2, 3, 4
7. 1, 3, 4, 5

(see page 138)

What Else Helps Pronation when Utilizing the Inverted Orthotic Technique

Discussion of what will help their bad flat feet is very helpful to have them understand not just to rely on the foot orthotic devices. Foot health is helped by changes in many factors. These factors should be part of their overall program. They include: functional foot orthotic devices, taping, strengthening exercises, stable shoes, high top boots occasionally, stretching when there are equinus forces, and gait changes. Foot health can also be dependent on how one abuses or respects their feet in exercise. The most common strengthening exercises include: posterior and anterior tibial tendons, peroneus longus tendon, intrinsic foot muscles with metatarsal doming, single leg balancing or single leg poses in yoga, tai chi, or qigong, 2 positional heel raises, lateral hamstrings and external hip rotators.

#29 Orthotic devices are commonly the only thing used when someone has pronated feet, but it should be part of an overall program of foot health. This program should include:
1. Functional Foot Orthotic Devices
2. Appropriate Strengthening Exercises
3. Appropriate Shoe Gear
4. Appropriate Changes in Gait Patterns
5. Appropriate Activity and Training Techniques
6. All of the above

(see page 138)

Follow Up Advice

Discussion of follow up is crucial to make sure that they are on board with all aspects of treatment. This type of medicine is vital to have follow up visits. The visits are to make sure that they are getting used to the orthotics, that they are progressing through their strengthening program, that they are resolving the equinus found, that their shoe selection has been great, and that they are overall feeling healthier and better. I personally like to follow my patients on a monthly basis and biomechanically no more than 3 aspects are being dealt with (otherwise none of them will be accomplished due to patient overload). Again, what are these components of treatment? They include custom or over the counter inserts (and perhaps just varus or valgus wedging), taping, lifts for short leg, shoe selections, weak muscles with strengthening, tight muscles with flexibility work, physical therapy with muscle work and gait changes, training patterns (like starting a walk run program), cross training (for cardio and strength), and new programs of Tai Chi, Pilates, etc.

#30 On follow up visits in biomechanics, you are trying to keep the pain level between 0-2 (a healing environment), as you make the patient more stable and stronger. The following can be very helpful in this regard.
1. Evaluate overall stability of orthotic devices and make recommendations for change if needed
2. Evaluate any tightness or muscle weakness

3. Evaluate how the patient is performing their exercises
4. Evaluate gait and the various shoes that they brought and make comments
5. Evaluate where their activity is and should be progressing towards
6. Evaluate any need of lifts, wedges, cushions or other simple mechanical changes
7. All of the above

(see page 138)

Break In Period

Discussion of break-in period is so vital to getting their bodies used to the significant change I am making. This is fully covered in Appendix 10. I will make this change in 2 years old to 92 years old if they need it. Children definitely adapt easier than my elderly patients, but it can be done. Functional foot orthotics should have a 1 hour per day increase in wearing for the first 10 days. The full body changes, especially with the Inverted Technique, can be significant. Running can start at 1 mile the first day, and progress a mile per workout every other day. The rule has to be no pain at any time in the progress.

#31 Which is not part of an orthotic break in period?
1. Hourly increases in time walking
2. Hourly increases in time any position
3. 1 mile increase every other day in runners
4. Blame any new ache or pain on the new orthotic devices
5. Modify the new orthotic devices when the patient first gets them for pain sensations, not unusual pressure sensations

(see page 138)

What Makes A Patient Stable

Discussion of what makes a patient biomechanically stable is so important. This is actually the same as what helps their bad feet. Overall, if I have a decision to make on treatment, which course to go, I always go towards greater stability. When the symptoms do not let me make a patient more stable, I always document why I had to compromise (like why I had to drop the medial arch, why I had to put motion in the rearfoot post, or why I felt the patient should have a soft based orthotic device over a plastic base). Typically in clinical practice you are continuously trying to make a patient more stable with a progression of the following:

1. Varus Wedges, OTC inserts, or custom made inserts
2. Shoe changes for more stability
3. Arch or ankle taping
4. Foot, ankle, and lower limb strengthening exercises
5. Stretching programs to help with any equinus forces found
6. Training programs to restart after injury or just overall more balanced program with more recovery times
7. Overall health issues including proper sleep, proper diet, bone health

I hope this book helps you go from a surgeon or orthotic maker to the guardian of the patient's foot health. You can feel almost like one of those Guardians of the Galaxy characters.

Manufacturing the Inverted Mold

http://www.drblakeshealingsole.com/search?q=inverted+orthotic+arch+height

The following is the step by step photos of the manufacturing process of one patient with a pair of 25 degree inverted orthoses for his running. The Inverted Orthotic Technique, other then when using the Fettig modification, will ignore the forefoot to rearfoot relationship, so it works on the rearfoot mechanics alone.

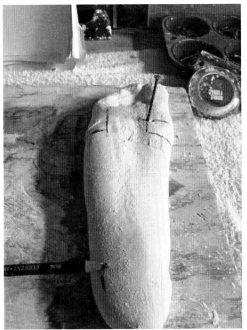

Lines for the 1st and 5th anterior platforms are made and then a nail under the first metatarsal head to give the amount of inversion (this case was 25 degrees)

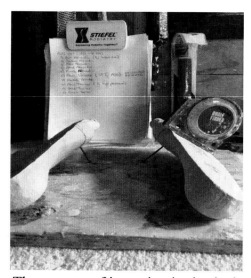

The amount of inversion is checked. Hopefully you can appreciate that for the same degrees of heel inversion needed, a bigger nail will be needed in a forefoot varus foot than a forefoot valgus type foot. This is one of the reasons I try to manipulate out any forefoot supinatus which is only soft tissue tightness anyway.

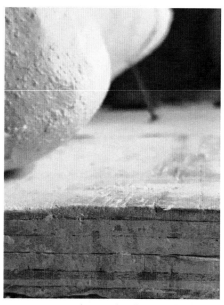

It is easy to see how the inversion force is made onto the medial heel area and into the proximal arch. You can also appreciate how the flatness of the heel will affect the inversion more than a rounded heel.

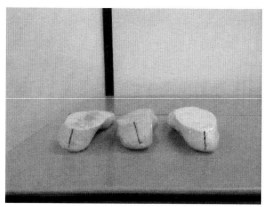

Here are 3 positive casts of the left foot with different forefoot deformities. I pour every cast vertical as my reference point. From right to left these casts represent a neutral forefoot, valgus (everted) forefoot, and varus (inverted) forefoot. If I set each one at 25 degrees inverted, the forefoot varus cast will need a bigger nail to get there.

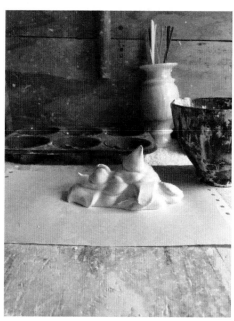

Plaster is laid down on paper to begin to make anterior platform which the biggest pile under the first metatarsal region.

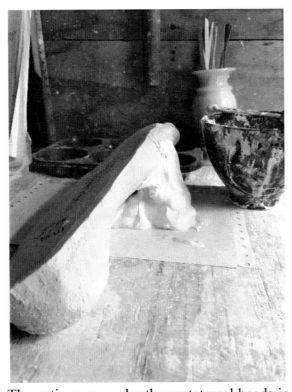

The entire area under the metatarsal heads is filled in and then smoothed to hold the inversion correction. It takes awhile to understand the right consistency of the plaster to mold well. The landmarks of the medial and lateral platforms are marked up each side to the top of the cast before the plaster work starts so that they can easily be found. It is important as soon as the anterior platform is made to check if it still represents the angle you wanted or you will have to remove and start again.

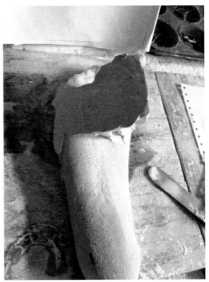

When first lifted off the table, the anterior platform with the 25 inversion, looks like this. I use all the plaster that I am going to remove as I square off the platform to begin the make the medial arch fill.

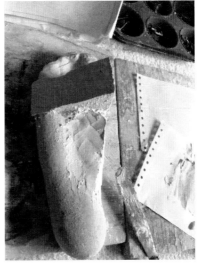

Then the anterior platform is squared off to the marked lines. The extra plaster begins to make the smooth arch fill and/or reinforce any weak spots noted on the anterior platform. As a laboratory technician, I am only skilled enough to do this process one foot at a time. But, in visiting many labs around the country, 5-10 feet at a time is quite common.

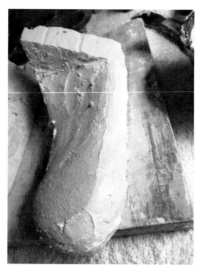

A lateral soft tissue expansion is applied roughly which should not involve the medial heel and not fill in the cuboid area. This expansion should be parallel with the anterior platform. It will next be straightened.

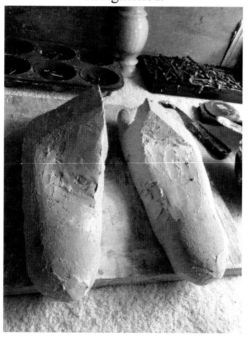

Beginnings of the important arch fill that should peak at the navicular 1st cuneiform joint and then gradually come down to the anterior platform which is the new supporting surface.

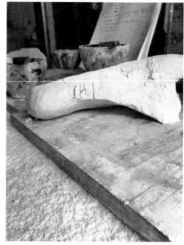

The rough "H" for the high point of the orthosis under the navicular 1st cuneiform and then tapered as it goes distally.

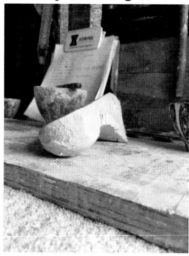

This view of the medial arch shows the inversion force at the rearfoot and the tapering away from the first ray to allow for plantar flexion. If I undercorrect patients with their initial orthosis by only 2-3 degrees, I can then apply a medial Kirby skive and slight medial column correction to this mold before I do a repress. The medial column correction is basically a smoothing of the Kirby into the "H" area so that there are no peaks that would be irritating to the wearer.

These following images are from a patient with a 35 degree inverted pair of orthotic devices.

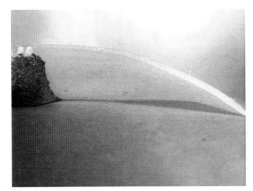

The distal aspect of the medial post should be flush with the anterior medial corner of the plastic. You can see how the highest peak of the medial arch is proximal at the 1st cuneiform navicular joint and then will fall away as it goes distally. The first metatarsal must be allowed to have an active plantarflexion at push off.

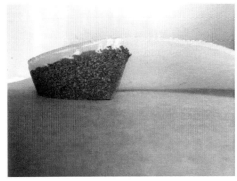

This photo emphasizes that the medial post should be firmly on the ground when the distal medial corner of the orthotic device is flush with the supporting surface. With many patients with high inversion, since I wanted a high medial heel cup (28 mm), I dropped the lateral heel cup to 23 mm for shoe fit (instead of 25 mm both sides for a standard 35 degree Inverted Device).

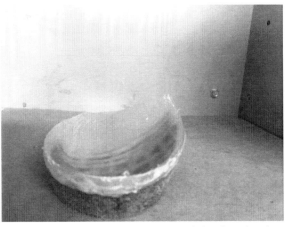

This posterior view of the finished orthotic device shows the medial heel support with the lateral heel cup and phalange.

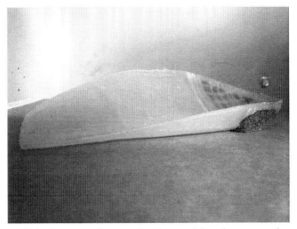

This image shows the lateral heel cup and phalange preventing lateral instability from the highly corrected 35 degree Inverted Orthotic Device.

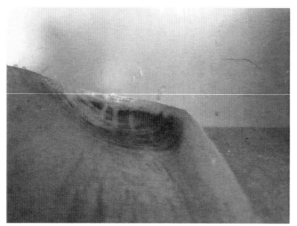

Another image of the lateral wall created to prevent lateral instability. The lateral area under the cuboid and 5th metatarsals are parallel with the ground (not inverted).

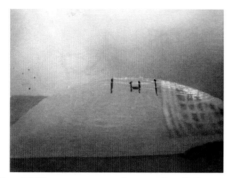

The "H" represents the peak of the arch under the first cuneiform navicular joint.

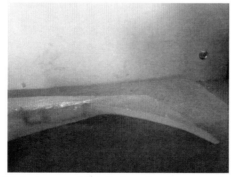

This image highlights the drop in the contour of the orthotic device above the first metatarsal to allow first metatarsal plantarflexion at heel lift.

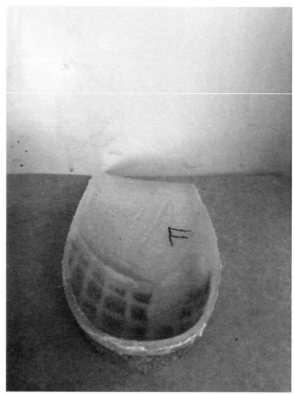

The "F" presents the Feehery cuboid support area. It is the area of the orthotic device that we need the most stability and the key to a stable lateral column.

#32 Which statement is false about the Inverted Orthotic Technique?

1. The height of the arch should peak superiorly under the first metatarsal base.
2. A plantar fascial groove should be built into every Inverted Orthotic Devices.
3. A Kirby Skive typically gives me 6 degrees of varus rearfoot correction.
4. More inversion force is generated by a round heel than a flat heel (that are then inverted).
5. All of the above
6. None of the above

(see page 138)

Conclusion

I hope this book will help in your understanding of the Inverted Orthotic Technique. The Appendices to follow will help improve the basic concepts like gait evaluation, symptoms improved with pronation control, other factors helpful to fight a pronation problem, and much more. I am hopeful that this book helps you and your orthotic laboratory understand this technique better and ultimately helps your patients. It has so many uses. I have doctors that I have consulted with only using them with runners, or only using them with Stage 2 and 3 posterior tibial tendon dysfunction, or only using them in pediatric flatfoot cases. I hope this book helps you broaden your scope of use, or simply to try it once when the right patient comes along. Encourage your orthotic laboratory to read this book and look at my videos and blog posts. The Inverted Orthotic Technique is my gift to my beloved profession, and this book is long overdue.

Appendix 1: Pain produced by over pronation

When utilizing the Inverted Orthotic Technique, you must be familiar with the symptoms of excessive pronation (and described next in Appendix 2 of excessive supination). A patient can come in for treatment for a foot and ankle injury, but also have a variety of other symptoms that may be helped with your orthotic devices. I have had patients who present with up to 10 issues at one time. If you treat this patient mechanically, it is great to see which symptoms are helped and which are not (and may need other forms of treatment). There may even be those symptoms made worse by your mechanical changes, and you may have to figure out a hybrid compromise. It can be an interesting process that the patients are normally so thankful for your help. I emphasize that the mechanical changes from any stabilizing orthotic device, especially the Inverted Orthotic Technique, can make a powerful change to the foot, ankle, leg, knee, hip and low back mechanics. Normally, if you make someone more stable, you will improve their physical and emotional health.

Here is a list I give to my students that can be caused by excessive pronation. The list was generated by various articles, but mainly years of evaluation of what symptoms could improve if I corrected for excessive pronation. The list for pronation is founded on the problems or instabilities produced by over pronation: medial instability, excessive rotation or torque on various structures, poor shock absorption if you are fully pronated, increased medial foot weight bearing, and lateral knee weight bearing. They include:

1. First metatarsal phalangeal joint pain with functional hallux limitus.
2. Sesamoid Injuries can be caused by pronation injuring the sesamoids.
3. Bunions are caused by the chronic nature of pronation overloading the medial side of the foot causes instability of the first metatarsal first cuneiform joint leading to slow first metatarsal drift in abduction, inversion, dorsiflexion.
4. Second metatarsal phalangeal joint capsulitis where an unstable 1st metatarsal puts more weight on the second metatarsal.
5. Metatarsalgia can be caused by the shearing forces of forefoot abduction on the rearfoot.
6. Second metatarsal stress fractures can be caused by the overload onto the 2nd metatarsal from an unstable 1st metatarsal.
7. Morton's neuromas or neuritis can be caused by instability of the metatarsals when the foot stays too pronated (loose bag of bones) and there is excessive intermetatarsal motion.
8. Hammertoes can be caused by lack of stability in the midfoot, so the toes claw the ground in an attempt to gain stability.
9. Intrinsic muscle strain occurs when the muscles have to work overtime

stabilizing the foot, especially the digits at propulsion.

10. Plantar fasciitis is an overstretching of the arch with pronation that probably is related to microtearing.

11. Anterior tibial tendonitis develops with excessive pronation and the attempt at decelerating that pronation at heel contact.

12. Lateral sinus tarsitis, also called sinus tarsi syndrome, is normally lateral impingement with marked eversion where the medial structures are stretched and the lateral structures pinched.

13. Cuboid syndrome is where the cuboid is not stable and the tissue around it get irritated. Excessive pronation means medial weight bearing, but lateral foot instability.

14. Lateral ankle impingement, like sinus tarsi syndrome, where high levels of pronation cause the everting calcaneus to collide with the medial side of the lateral malleolus.

15. Posterior tibial injuries including accessory navicular syndrome. The posterior tibial tendon is the most important and most direct decelerator of subtalar joint pronation and supporter on the medial longitudinal arch.

16. Tarsal tunnel syndrome can have a mechanical cause or aggravating factor where pronation of the foot at the ankle can cause a stretching of the medial ankle structures for a prolonged or exaggerated timeframe. Also, swelling from tenosynovitis of any of the three medial ankle tendons can cause posterior tibial nerve compression.

17. Peroneus longus strain can occur from overpronation where the tendon attempts to stabilize the medial column where it attaches.

18. Achilles strain can occur from overpronation as the achilles medial fibers fight to decelerate pronation. The achilles is a sagittal plane mover primarily, and can get stressed and twisted when the heel is everted to the tibial during push off from overpronation.

19. Tibial stress fractures can be caused by overpronation causes excessive internal tibial rotation. Some of the biggest muscles that decelerate this pronation attach on the tibia called the posterior tibial and soleus. The pull can be so great that the tibia can break. Since knee motion can be dependent or independent on foot motion, there are many individuals that have tremendous foot pronation with no patellar internal rotation. In these situations, the torque that naturally goes up the leg into the knee and hip, is stopped in the tibia or knee abruptly leading to tibial stress.

20. Medial soleus strain can be caused with overpronation. The soleus attaches into both the proximal aspects on the posterior tibia and posterior fibula. It not only works to plantar flex the ankle at push off, but supinates the subtalar joint to help

with the overall external leg rotation of the lower extremity. If the foot is held in a prolonged pronated position into the propulsive phase, or if the foot pronates in the late midstance or propulsive phases, the soleus fibres can stress and muscle strain occurs.

21. Lateral knee compartment injury can be produced with overpronation. If you have lateral meniscal issues, you would want to open up and decompress the lateral compartment by varus wedging the foot. But, the knee joint is influenced by foot motion, the knee's own axis of motion, and by hip motion. Therefore, 50% of patients do not respond to lateral wedging, but everyone seemed to be helped by some form of foot stability correction.

22. Pes anserinus tendinitis/bursitis can be produced by overpronation. The 3 muscles that make up the pes anserinus attach into the proximal medial aspect of the anterior tibia for stabilization at foot contact of the knee. The three muscles are the sartorius, gracilis, and semitendinosus also called guy ropes. By their attachment, at foot strike, and it is primarily a running related injury, it stabilizes the anterior medial knee area which is stressed in the overpronation motion of excessive internal tibial rotation on the femur. It protects the anterior cruciate ligament which is trying to stop the anterior and medial displacement of the tibia on the femur from inside the knee. I especially see it in downhill running, where these medial knee structures have to stabilize a flexing knee at foot strike where the force can be 10 times body weight.

23. Patellofemoral injuries can be produced by overpronation. The problem lies in the kneecap or patella not staying in its normal femoral groove, but sliding laterally thus irritating the medial aspect of the posterior surface of the patella. This lateral subluxation is helped with taping the patella slightly medially, bracing the patella to hold it more centered, strengthening the vastus medialis and external hip rotators, and stretching the very powerful vastus lateralis to weaken its pull laterally. With overpronation, sometimes just produced by the sport in a normal foot, 2 mechanisms can be to blame either fully or partially. If the overpronation causes the knee to assume a more valgus position of the tibia on the femur, this alignment causes the vastus lateralis to have more power pulling the patella laterally. If the overpronation simply produces more internal rotation of the tibia on the femur, the vastus lateralis is placed in tone, and the vastus medialis relaxed creating a dynamic muscle imbalance leading again to the lateral subluxation of the patella.

24. Anterior Cruciate Injuries can be helped by pronation correction. I do not think that ACL injuries are caused by overpronation, but from our previous discussion of pes anserinus injuries, the anterior cruciate ligament functions to stop both anterior motion of the tibia on the femur and internal rotation of the tibia on the femur. When treating patients with ACL injuries, either conservatively or post operatively, custom orthotics or simply varus wedges that can control the internal rotation of the tibia on the femur can take a great deal of stress away from the ACL.

25. Medial hamstring strains can be produced by overpronation. The medial hamstrings are the semimembranosus, attaching into the posterior medial aspect of the proximal tibia, and the semitendinosus, attaching into the anterior medial aspect of the proximal tibia. In normal function, the medial hamstrings are knee flexors and internal rotators of the tibia helping with foot pronation. However, with excessive foot pronation, the role of the semitendinosus as part of the pes anserinus must be to protect the anterior medial knee and stop the forward motion of the tibia. This repeated motion can cause strain of the medial hamstrings.

26. Iliotibial band syndrome can be caused by a variety of abnormal motions, and one of them is overpronation. The Iliotibial Band is one of my most favorite structures. Its primary function is to protect the lateral hip and the lateral knee at foot strike. It is prone to get tight, making it easier to strain. It is a very common running injury and it does not take a lot to cause it to be overworked. Excessive pronation is only one motion that can irritate it, but probably the most publicized. As the femur internally rotates with excessive subtalar joint pronation, the tibia, where the iliotibial band attaches, internally rotates more. This motion of internal rotation of the tibia on the femur brings the iliotibial band anterior over two body landmarks. These landmarks are the greater trochanters around the hip area and the lateral femoral epicondyles at the knee. Women typically develop ITBS at the hips and men at the knees.

27. Piriformis syndrome can be caused by overpronation. With walking and running, the piriformis is an external hip rotator. Therefore, excessive pronation which causes excessive internal hip rotation strains the piriformis muscle trying to decelerate that internal motion. The interesting and perplexing aspect of piriformis syndrome is how it can involve the sciatic nerve and cause neurological symptoms. The sciatic nerve can run under, over, or between the fibres of the piriformis.

So many problems we treat have a neuropathic aspect because the sciatic nerve gets irritated. You can get classic sciatica symptoms, or just vague neuropathic symptoms.

Checklist of Pronation Produced Problems:
1. First MPJ Pain
2. Sesamoid Pain
3. Bunions
4. Second MPJ Pain
5. Metatarsalgia
6. Second Metatarsal Stress Fracture
7. Morton's Neuroma/Neuritis
8. Hammertoes
9. Intrinsic Muscle Strain
10. Plantar Fasciitis
11. Anterior Tibial Strains
12. Sinus Tarsi Syndrome
13. Cuboid Syndrome
14. Lateral Ankle Impingement
15. Posterior Tibial Strains
16. Tarsal Tunnel Syndrome
17. Peroneus Longus Strains
18. Achilles Strains
19. Tibial Stress Fractures
20. Medial Soleus Strains
21. Lateral Knee Compartment Pain
22. Pes Anserinus Tendinitis/Bursitis
23. Patellofemoral Joint Pain
24. ACL support when injured
25. Medial Hamstring Strains
26. Iliotibial Band Strains
27. Piriformis Syndrome

#33 Which of the following is false regarding the pronation syndrome?

1. Pronation can inflame the piriformis as it tries to decelerate internal femoral rotation.
2. Pronation causes the iliotibial band tract to move posteriorly over the lateral femoral condyle.
3. Pronation causes part of the medial hamstring to overwork protecting the ACL.
4. Pronation can sprain the ACL as it attempts to protect the anterior medial knee joint area.

(see page 132)

#34 Which of the following statements are true?

1. Excessive Pronation leads to Runner's Knee as the patella moves out of its femoral groove medially.
2. Excessive Pronation stresses the pes anserinus as the anterior medial knee is stressed in running. The fibres of the pes anserinus are made up of the gracilis, sartorius, and semimembranosus.
3. Excessive Pronation in forefoot varus patients can cause compression stress to the lateral knee joint compartment.
4. Shin Splints caused by over pronation typically is produced by the lateral soleus fibres attempting to hold the heel vertical.

(see Appendix 12)

#35 Circle which injuries below can be related to excessive pronation.

1. Fibular stress fractures
2. Achilles strains
3. Peroneus brevis strain

4. Tarsal Tunnel Syndrome
5. Posterior Tibial Tendon Injuries

(see page 138)

#36 Which of the following is related to over pronation?
1. Anteromedial Ankle Impingement
2. Cuboid Syndrome
3. Medial Sinus Tarsitis
4. Intrinsic Foot Muscle Strain
5. 1,3,4
6. 2,4
7. All of the above

(see page 138)

#37 Overpronation can put a strain on the plantar fascia by causing an over-stretch problem. What is the weakest point for the stressed plantar fascia in the gait cycle?
1. Heel Strike
2. Forefoot Loading
3. Middle of Midstance
4. Heel Lift
5. Push Off

(see page 138)

Appendix 2: Pain produced by over supination

When utilizing the Inverted Orthotic Technique, you are changing a patient from someone who is:

1. In a too pronated position
2. Or, pronating excessively (this motion can be defined as too much, too fast, or at the wrong time).

This change produces the following at various times:

1. Less pronated position towards their ideal (neutral) position (still with an everted heel or vertical heel in resting stance).
2. Less pronated pronated position towards their ideal position (heel now inverted or more inverted as in tibial varum cases).
3. Less pronated position but now inverted from their ideal position.
4. Excessive supination at heel contact (also called lateral instability) which has to be reversed.

This position/movement change from pronation to supination can lead to symptoms. These symptoms are supinatory and can be temporary (just needing to get used to the new biomechanics) or more serious needing orthotic adjustments towards less pronation correction. They may be easily observed in gait, or very subtle like a patient feeling a slight lateral slide of their foot on the orthosis. You need to be aware of symptoms caused by too much supination when prescribing and working with patients with the Inverted Orthotic Technique.

Here is the list I give to students on the injuries created by excessive supination, which is also called under pronation, and also called lateral instability. Someone may be an excessive supinator only when they wear certain shoes. Someone may be structured to overly supinate even barefoot. Excessive supination causes injuries because of the lateral instability, because the lack of heel contact pronation means no shock absorption, because there is lateral weight bearing on the foot for a prolonged time, and there is excessive medial loading of the knee. Injuries can also occur since there is knee extension at contact, not the normal knee flexion. These injuries include:

1. Hammertoes due to the instability (abnormal supination is the most unstable situation the foot has to try to stabilize. A common way to attempt more foot stability is by clawing of the toes which can lead to hammertoe deformities. High arched feet with a normal increased metatarsal declination are already prone to hammertoe development. If you add supination instability to a high arched foot, the chance of development of hammertoes is around 100%).
2. Lateral metatarsalgia (abnormal supination typically occurs in contact phase of gait, but can linger throughout midstance into propulsion. This causes an overload of the lateral forefoot with lateral metatarsalgia symptoms developing. The treatment can be complicated since orthotic corrections for this

lateral overload sometimes requires the most force be placed on the sore area).

3. Tailor's bunion pain and development (tailor's bunions on the fifth metatarsal head are so much less complained about as normal first metatarsal bunions. One of the causes of tailors bunions is this lateral forefoot overload due to excessive supination which produces a chronic subluxation on the cuboid-fifth metatarsal joint articulation. The fifth ray motion when overloaded plantarly is towards eversion, abduction, and dorsiflexion. The abduction of the 5th metatarsal leads to a widening of the 5th ray and the obvious appearance of the tailor's bunion).

4. 4th and/or 5th metatarsal fractures (excessive supination causes lateral overload of the 4th and 5th metatarsals which both articulate with the cuboid. When that overload is fairly rapid (say in training too quickly for a marathon), either the 4th metatarsal or the 5th metatarsal may develop a stress fracture. A lot depends on the ability of these 2 metatarsals to move superiorly in reaction to the ground forces. They will always move differently and sometimes the fifth metatarsal moves upward enough that the fourth metatarsal takes the weight. Typically, most patients have a slight plantar flexed fifth metatarsal that takes the excessive weight and develops stress fractures likes a Jones fracture).

5. Cuboid pain from overload (excessive supination causing lateral overload on the cuboid and then some form of joint dysfunction and ensuing pain. Just after heel contact, the powerful gastroc-soleus complex contracts to push the cuboid towards the supporting surface. This produces a very stable midfoot and a key element in re-supination of the foot. With over supination, that cuboid loading goes too far, and depending what ligaments are loose, the cuboid is dorsiflexed possibly across various joints: calcaneocuboid, cuboid-third cuneiform, cuboid-4th or 5th metatarsals, or cuboid-navicular. This is opposite of cuboid syndrome post inversion ankle sprain where the cuboid gets stuck plantarly. The famous cuboid whip is designed to dorsiflex (or superiorly translate) the cuboid when stuck below its normal position).

6. Lateral ankle instability (excessive supination at contact phase is also called lateral instability. It is a disastrous motion when it occurs robbing the foot of shock absorption and placing an extension force on the knee when it should be flexing. Yet, it is the lateral stress at the ankle that can cause some of the most dangerous issues. When you combine this lateral foot and ankle instability with an unstable shoe or

unstable terrain or in the presence of old sprains, the patient may be set up for chronic issues. Lateral ankle instability is then brought on by injuries produced by the subtalar supination, or the instability caused by these injuries can cause more excessive supination. The pain from lateral ankle instability then can be acute when a new injury occurs, or chronic in all the areas excessive supination causes pain even the lateral or medial ankle areas).

7. Peroneal strain (excessive subtalar joint supination stresses the lateral side of the foot and ankle and one of the ways the body tries to protect itself is by excessively contracting the peroneal tendons. It can be both or more the peroneus longus or the peroneus brevis. It may be weak peroneal tendons that can not react without pain if the foot is in an unstable lateral position or motion. Like the complexity of the posterior tibial or all of the extrinsic ankle muscles, straining the peroneals can give you pain from its origin on the fibula to the insertions on the first (peroneus longus) or fifth (peroneus brevis) metatarsals or anywhere in between. I warn patients who have pain around the lateral malleolus and get an MRI that the tendons can look torn on MRI and be totally strong and non painful in examination).

8. Haglund's deformity and pain (the posterior superior lateral corner of the calcaneus is closer to the heel counter of shoes than the medial corner, and therefore will take more friction or stress from that interaction. Excessive supination at heel contact will magnify that lateral pressure on the posterior corner. Correction of the lateral rotation of excessive supination does 2 very positive things to the Haglund's bump aka retrocalcaneal exostosis or pump bump. The first function of an orthotic device is in minimizing the lateral drift of the heel therefore decreasing the force that creates or irritates the deformity. The second function of the orthotic device is in simply raising the heel slightly so that there is less pressure in the same area).

9. Medial ankle impingement (excessive supination affects the talus by moving it medially within the ankle mortise to crowd the medial talar dome and medial talar border on the lateral surface of the medial malleolus. If that inversion is sudden, like in an inversion ankle sprain, bony injury can occur to the talus or tibia. If the inversion is less forceful, but consistent, as in activities of repetitive motion like walking, hiking, biking, etc, the soft tissue can get irritated. When I make orthotics for patients, even Root Balanced, I can create an inversion force too much that leads to medial ankle impingement. This is very common when the patient is fine until the shoe starts to break down

laterally increasing the inversion force across all joints).

10. Fibular stress fractures (excessive subtalar joint supination increases lateral weight bearing in the foot, but that weight bearing stress goes medially into the talus and tibia as just described, not the fibula. The excessive supination affects the fibula by producing an unstable lateral ankle which compensates with tremendous muscle pull of the peroneals. The pull can be so stressful that it breaks the fibula by muscle contraction only. I once treated a semi-professional ballet dancer that sickled (excessive supination in ballet terms) en pointe. The teacher had been trying to correct this technique error, but she broke her fibula 3 different times in the course of 2 years. Finally, both better technique and a think sewn thread along the lateral border of the end of her pointe shoe fixed the problem).

11. Proximal tib-fib sprain (excessive supination increases the medial weight bearing across the knee joint and opens up the lateral joint capsule. This can be used in cases of lateral meniscal tears, either post operatively to decompress the lateral compartment or in an attempt to avoid surgery in non bucket handle tears, by adding varus wedges or inversion forces into custom orthotic devices. However, in opening up the lateral capsule of the knee, you are also causing instability at the proximal tib-fib joint which can get grade 1 sprain symptoms).

12. Medial knee compartment overload (excessive supination overloads the medial knee joint. Medial knee meniscus problems and degenerative joint problems plague society. It is a problem of knee extension, whereas societies that bend that knees more get lateral meniscus issues. The patient presents with pain, and sometimes swelling, along the medial knee joint line).

13. Knee arthralgias (excessive supination jars the knees by robbing the foot of its shock absorption through contact phase pronation. Correcting the supination can soften the knees at impact, even when using a plastic device. Since deep knee pain can present in various ways, sometimes very hard to localize, it may be the medial knee compartment overload syndrome just presenting more generalized).

14. Lateral collateral ligament sprain (excessive supination opens the lateral knee joint line and can sprain the lateral collateral ligament attaching to the head of the fibula).

15. Lateral hamstring strain (excessive supination opens up the lateral joint line being protected by the lateral hamstrings attaching into the head of the fibula. The lateral hamstrings may be strained for this function. The hamstrings themselves are knee joint flexors, whereas excessive

supination puts an extension force on the knee when it should be flexing. This may strain the hamstrings. With this extension force at the knee, there can be more jarring. The hamstrings may strain in attempt to flex the knee thereby relaxing the tension within the knee joint itself).

16. Iliotibial band syndrome (excessive supination of the foot causes lateral instability affecting the soft tissues that guard the whole lateral one half of our extremities. I have talked about the effect on the peroneal tendons and hamstrings, but the iliotibial band is probably the most affected. The iliotibial band functions to protect the lateral side of the hip and the lateral side of the knee at foot strike. It is a common running injury since the force that needs to be stabilized can be 7 times that of walking, and running mechanics tend naturally to be more inverted for longer times. Excessive supination of the foot on top of all these other factors can easily lead to an overload of the iliotibial band as it tries to protect the hip and knee).

17. Femoral stress fractures (excessive supination robs the body of its foot shock absorption leading to increase stress up the leg. Excessive supination also causes knee extension at foot strike accentuating jarring forces at the knee and hip. Femoral stress fractures in relatively young patients is seen in runners where the athlete has to absorb up to 7 times body weight while downhill running. If you add low Vitamin D, inadequate diet issues, shoes that have broken down recently, or some combination of factors, and a tendency to supinate, it is easy to imagine the femur developing stress reactions and fractures).

18. Hip arthralgias (excessive supination robs the body of needed shock absorption and can cause increased joint loading at the knee, hip, and sacroiliac joints).

19. Sacroiliac joint inflammation from upward jamming (the sacroiliac joint is a gliding joint that primarily moves in the sagittal plane both inferiorly and superiorly. When the heel contacts the ground and the knee is straight, that can drive up the ilium on the stationary sacrum. The SI joint is said to be stuck superiorly and symptoms can occur. If you have ever misjudged the height of a step and landed with a jerk, the sacroiliac joint takes that force and can be placed in the wrong position causing joint symptoms. Excessive subtalar joint supination extends the knee and can force this scenario more insidiously from repetitive motion. The patient is then unaware of a cause but complains of chronic back pain).

20. Low back pain from poor shock absorption or excessive hamstring pull (we know that our hamstrings are tighter when we straighten the knee, and looser when we bend our

knee. As we straighten the knee from excessive supination, this puts more of a stretch on the hamstrings and gastrocnemius that both cross the back of the knee joint. The hamstrings attach into the ischial tuberosities (sit bones). This tension in the hamstrings pulls down on the pelvis to extend the hip at a time in gait when the hip should be flexing. This extension force on the hip and pelvis also straightens our back causing muscle and disc irritations).

Checklist for Supination Produced Problems
1. Hammertoes
2. Lateral Metatarsalgia
3. Tailor's Bunions
4. 4th/5th Metatarsal Stress Fractures
5. Cuboid Pain
6. Lateral Ankle Instability
7. Peroneal Strain
8. Haglund's Deformity
9. Medial Ankle Impingement
10. Fibular Stress Fractures
11. Proximal Tib-Fib Sprain
12. Medial Knee Compartment
13. Knee Arthralgias
14. Lateral Knee Collateral Ligament Sprain
15. Lateral Hamstring Strain
16. Iliotibial Band Syndrome
17. Femoral Stress Fractures
18. Hip Arthralgias
19. Sacroiliac joint inflammation
20. Low Back Pain

#38 Understanding lower extremity biomechanics can help patients with lower back pain. Excessive rearfoot supination at heel contact can cause low back pain due to the following:
1. Excessive knee flexion
2. Excessive knee extension
3. Excessive knee internal rotation
4. Inadequate limb shock absorption
5. 1 and 3
6. 2 and 4

(see page 138)

#39 When a patient is observed with excessive supination at heel contact, what symptoms can not be tied to that abnormal out of phase motion?
1. Sacro-iliacitis
2. Femoral stress fractures
3. Fibular stress fractures
4. Lateral knee compartment
5. Peroneal tendon strain
6. 4th or 5th metatarsal stress fracture

(see page 138)

#40 When a patient has excessive subtalar joint supination, it is called:
1. Lateral Instability
2. Under Pronation
3. Excessive Lateral Weight Bearing
4. All of the above

(see page 138)

#41 Excessive contact phase supination is known for its lateral lower extremity problems as a general rule, whereas pronation is known for its medial problems. What medial problems are associated with this lateral instability?
1. Medial knee compartment pain

2. Peroneus longus insertional tendinitis
3. Os tibial externum syndrome
4. Medial ankle arthralgias
5. All of the above
6. 1 and 4 only

(see page 138)

#42 Excessive supination can be related to foot function only (ie. plantar flexed first ray), shoe function only (ie. 4 inch high heels with worn heel), or a combination of both. When the over supination is related to shoe function, what are some of the components of the shoes seen in the office that leads to this?

1. High Heel type of shoe
2. Excessive medial heel support
3. Inadequate lateral heel or midfoot support
4. Excessive lateral heel wear
5. Very cushioning shoe
6. All of the above

(see page 138)

#43 Biomechanics is all about stresses. We have different stresses with different environments. Varying shoes, varying orthotic devices, and varying training patterns to name a few of these variables, can help prevent injury. If you do not change the patient's oversupination, what are some ways you can still help them?

1. Change shoe types every 3rd workout
2. Change training patterns to less stressful
3. Change heel strike patterns based on injury type

4. Strengthen musculature to decelerate supination (like the peroneals)
5. All of the above

(see page 138)

#44 Our lower extremity joints are the most stable when centered or stacked under each other at the middle of the midstance phase of gait. If that alignment of the foot to ankle has the weight bearing too medial with an inverted heel, it is called oversupination. The weight of the ankle and knee is too medial, but the weight in the foot is too lateral. Between this inverted heel and excessive lateral foot weight bearing, the peroneal tendons get stressed. What are the common reasons for peroneal tendonitis?

1. Excessive Supination
2. Peroneal Weakness
3. Acute Injury following an Ankle Sprain
4. Chronic Fatigue due to unstable shoes
5. All of the above

(see page 138)

Appendix 3: 12 Point Biomechanical Outline

The following is a nice office outline you can follow seeing patients. You start with the history of the injury, overall health status like Vitamin D deficiency and inflammatory conditions, and past injury history. You then watch them walk and/or run, and try to correlate the injury to their biomechanics (this may have to wait several visits due to their injury). You then break down the physical examination to mechanical problems, inflammation, and possible neuropathic problems. Based on your tentative diagnosis, your examination gets more specific. You also look at the area for possible biomechanical factors affecting it (the better you are at biomechanics, the more you can probe deeply like checking equinus with any metatarsal problem). Then, you start to focus on the asymmetry of the problem and how to address that (like the weaker side or the more pronated side). After you have made your tentative diagnosis, begin to apply your Occam's Law (the most obvious cause is probably the cause) and the Rule of 3 (most injuries require 3 causes to occur or be fixed for healing and overall injury prevention).

It is important in medicine to have the opportunity to second guess ourselves. This is the role of the common differential diagnosis, our second choice of a diagnosis if the tentative diagnosis proves wrong. This is developing a Plan B when Plan A doesn't work out. There is hope in this scenario. From there, we then have to decide what Phase of Rehabilitation the patient fits into at the time. And we have to decide on whether imaging is important or can potentially wait for a while.

Finally, we have to develop our plan to get the pain down to 0-2 over the shortest time possible with mechanical, inflammatory, and neuropathic treatments. I typically see my patients monthly for injuries, making sure they progress through the process, and helping them with plateaus and setbacks. This checklist is a wonderful help for any visit along this journey.

1. History affecting cause and overall health status_____

_____

_____

_____

_____

_____

2. Finding on Gait important to Injury or just unique to patient_____

_____

_____

_____

_____

_____

_____

3. Finding on Physical Examination (in particular signs of mechanical, inflammatory, neuropathic)_____

_____

_____

_____

_____
_____

4. Findings specific for the general and localized injury area biomechanics_____

_____
_____
_____
_____

5. Is there Asymmetry?_____

_____
_____
_____

6. What is the tentative diagnosis?

_____
_____
_____
_____

7. What is Occam's Law for this diagnosis? Does the Rule of 3 apply?_____

_____
_____
_____
_____
_____
_____

8. What is the most common differential diagnosis (different than the tentative diagnosis)?_____

_____
_____
_____

9. What Phase of Rehabilitation applies today?_____

_____

10. Should we Image today?_____

_____

11. How will 0-2 Pain Levels be Obtained? Mechanical Measures? Anti-Inflammatory Measures? Neuropathic Measures?_____

_____
_____
_____
_____

12. What is our Mechanical Treatment today?_____

_____
_____
_____
_____

Checklist for Biomechanical Visit
  1. History
  2. Gait Findings
  3. Physical Examination
  4. Biomechanical Findings
  5. Asymmetry?
  6. Tentative Diagnosis
  7. Occam's Law and Rule of 3?
  8. Differential Diagnosis
  9. Phase of Rehabilitation
  10. Imaging?
  11. How to attain 0-2 Pain Level?
  12. Mechanical Treatment Today

#45 Functional asymmetry is a big concept utilized in the treatment of the Inverted Orthotic Technique. Most patients are asymmetrical for various reasons including whether they are right or left handed.

Treating each side differently is so important to get lower leg function closer to symmetrical patterns. The following is not a reason patients present with asymmetrical function:

1. Short Leg Syndrome
2. Previous Past Injuries
3. Weak Left Posterior Tibial or Piriformis Tendons.
4. Previous Surgery Lower Extremity
5. Unilateral Tibial Varum
6. None of the Above

(see page 138)

#46 Match up the following with the Phases of Rehabilitation.

1. Theraband Progressive Resistance
2. Prednisone Burst
3. Cam Walker
4. Walk Run Program
5. 4 Straight Days of Icing
6. Active Range of Motion or Isometric Exercises

(see page 138)

#47 Occam's Law does not match up with which one of the following.

1. Tight Achilles and Achilles Tendonitis
2. Morton's Neuromas and Tight Shoes
3. Bunions and Tight Shoes
4. Ankle Sprain and Forefoot Varus Deformity
5. Iliotibial Band Syndrome and Over Pronation

(see page 138)

#48 What level of pain is needed to allow a patient heal from most injuries?

1. 4-5
2. 2-3
3. 0-2
4. 1-4
5. 3-5

(see page 138)

#49 What are the 3 general types of pain you need to treat, especially in chronic injuries?

_____

(see page 138)

Appendix 4: Gait Evaluation and Symptoms

In my training, gait evaluation was a crucial part in assessing how the inserts worked in controlling excessive motion, correcting for a short leg, improving someone's posture, but also spotting problems. These problems could be very obvious like limping from pain or more subtle like a twist in the foot at propulsion from abnormal pronation. And I have had my share of patients over the years who stated my findings on gait evaluation lead to the proper diagnosis of a neurological disease and the proper treatment. Even though a thorough understanding of structural deviations is vital to our training as taught with Root Biomechanics, gait evaluation really became my key to unraveling why someone hurt and sometimes where they hurt. In gait evaluation, you should look for signs of excessive pronation or supination or both (called medial-lateral instability), signs of short leg syndrome, signs of poor shock absorption, signs of limping and tight muscles, signs of weak muscles or instabilities, and signs of obvious structural problems like bow legs, knock knees, tibial varum, genu valgum, high arches, etc. You never waste anyone's time doing gait evaluations, and no one else seems to be doing it. I also had a patient tell me after 4 years of unsuccessful treatment that my gait evaluation was the only thing that unlocked the answer to their particular problem and the cure. Am I a believer?

So, where do we begin? When you watch someone walk, even from a podiatrist's standpoint, you want to start at the top. You need the patient in shorts, with their shirt tucked in, not looking down at their feet or walking slower than normal. You want them to walk 5 to 10 times up and down the longest hallway you can access so that they can get into a normal stride. Typically, if they have orthotic devices, I watch them walk with shoes and their orthotic devices first, then shoes tied up tightly without their orthotic devices. I want to see the difference in gait with and without their present orthotic devices. Then I will watch them walk barefoot to check any differences from shoe walking. Some people are more stable with shoes than barefoot, and some the opposite. Sometimes the most stable environment is barefoot, with shoes second, and shoes with orthotic devices third. You have to look and make observations. You are a scientist making observations. Try to throw away general rules, since there are so many exceptions. Some orthotic devices take a slight adjustment to make better, some need to be redone. Some patients only need to learn power lacing, also called runners knot or stability lacing. Sometimes patients just come in with very poor shoes, and proper evaluation of the function of orthotic devices will not occur until they purchase a better shoe. I also like to have patients bring in 2-4 pairs of shoes, especially some with a lot of wear, so I can see how they break down their shoes.

#50 What factors are not part of typical gait evaluation?

1. Comparison of orthotic devices to no orthotic devices

2. Looking at what environment the patient is the most stable
3. Starting at the feet for clues of stability
4. One walk down a long hallway should be enough
5. Never watch a patient barefoot, since they are never barefoot in real life for more than a few seconds

(see page 138)

Checklist for Gait Evaluation (circle findings)

1. Head Tilt (Right or Left)
2. Shoulder Drop
3. Asymmetrical Arm Swing
4. Dominance to One Side
5. Limited Trunk Mobility vs. Excessive Trunk Mobility
6. Hip Hike (Right or Left)
7. Higher Belt Line (Right or Left)
8. Hip Rotation (limited, normal, excessive)
9. Excessive Shock (Right or Left or Both)
10. Limited Knee Rotation(Right—straight vs external, Left—straight vs external)
11. Excessive Internal Knee Rotation (Right or Left or Both)
12. Subtalar Joint Motion at Heel Contact (Right—eversion, none, inversion, Left—eversion, none, inversion)
13. Arch Collapse (Right or Left or Both)
14. Symmetry of Arch Collapse (Right more vs Left more)
15. Digital Clawing (Right or Left or Both)
16. Angle of Gait (Right—internal, straight, external, Left—internal, straight, external)
17. Other Structural Observations: Pes Cavus, Pes Planus, Tibial Varum, Genu Valgum, etc
18. Correlation to Symptoms and other observations:

_____
_____
_____
_____
_____
_____
_____

#51 In the big picture, which of the following problems can be picked up in gait evaluation?
1. Signs of Short Leg Syndrome
2. Signs of Excessive Pronation
3. Signs of Excessive Supination
4. Signs of Poor Shock Absorption
5. Signs of Weak Muscles
6. Signs of Tight Muscles
7. All of the Above

(see page 138)

Signs of Possible Short Leg Syndrome

Common Signs of Short Leg Syndrome
1. Limb Dominance where the patient spends more of their time over one side
2. Asymmetrical arm swing (long leg can have the arm closer to the body)

3. Shoulder drop is usually on the long side
4. Head tilt is usually to the long side
5. More pronation or more supination on one side
6. Belt height is angled up towards one side

Since gait evaluation starts at the head, it is appropriate to begin our examination looking for signs of short leg syndrome. Short leg syndrome is actually divided into structural, where one leg is actually shorter, functional, where one hip is lower not due to shorter bones, and combination leg length discrepancy due to both structure and function. With a structural short leg, the femur or the tibia or both are shorter on one side. This can be very important in bike fitting. With functional (like a chronic bent knee post surgery), the hips are still dropped and havoc is played out on the pelvis and back. I focus on the low back as a podiatrist, but I know the entire spine and shoulders are affected with curves to compensate for unevenness of the hips and pelvis and sacral base (where the spine sits on top of the sacrum). Physiatrists, at least those trained in the EU, view the sacral base unevenness in a Standing AP Pelvis x-ray as the most important finding. As the spine twists and compensates, uneven tightness and weakness set up on both sides of the spine, and discs are compressed more on one side with the development of various neural tension areas. And, this can simply start as a child with one foot more pronated than the other, or following an ankle sprain, one side functions more supinated. Pronation drops the arch, whereas supination lifts up the

arch. Pronation drops the hip socket, supination lifts up the hip socket. This asymmetry causes unevenness which causes problems to develop. What are the common signs of short leg syndrome, also called limb length discrepancy, also called leg length difference? They include:

1. Head Tilt from the cervical tilt
2. Dropped Shoulder with lower fingers on that side
3. Asymmetrical Arm Swing '
4. Dropped Belt or Waist Line
5. Lean to one side (Dominance) which can vary in gait evaluation

#52 Which statements are false in leg length discrepancies?
1. The typical limb dominance is to the long leg
2. A true shoulder drop finding has lower fingers on that side
3. The more pronated side is the shorter side
4. The Standing AP Pelvis x-ray without lifts is the most important x-ray

(see page 138)

Signs of Excessive Pronation

Common Signs of Excessive Pronation
1. Internal rotation at the knees is excessive
2. The medial prominence of the ankle
3. Digital clawing in midstance
4. Abductory twist seen in propulsion
5. Heel eversion is sometimes seen
6. Arch collapse is noticeable as the patient walks toward you

I have spent my whole podiatric life correcting for overpronation, so I may be ready for another problem. I have had exposure to many orthotic laboratories, and this is the motion they excel at treating. What is it? Excessive Pronation means that there is foot motion of heel eversion at heel contact, medial foot adduction towards the other foot, arch collapse, and first metatarsal dorsiflexion is excessive (observed by functional hallux limitus in the stance evaluation). By excessive, we mean that the foot may be moving too far inward towards the other foot, or for too long a time period past contact phase into midstance or propulsion when the foot should be supinating, or that the pronation is just too fast producing a jerk on the system. But, it can also imply, that the foot is rigid in a fully pronated position as in a rigid flatfoot (to me this qualifies for poor shock absorption, but this fully pronated position can be poorly aligned with the rest of the joints). We need pronation for shock absorption as we make contact with the ground. We do not want it to be too much, too fast, at the wrong time, or ending up putting our bodies in abnormal positions. When I watch people walk or run, or bike, or dance, etc, I look for signs that the body is not lined up right. When the body is not lined up right, the foot is not centered under the ankle, the knee is over towards the other foot too much, or just a flat foot flopping along with poor body alignment and no shock absorption. This is not just a walking problem, but a problem with most repetitive motion sports. The mechanics for most of these sports have basic similar needs of effective sagittal plane motion, not too much

transverse and frontal plane drifts, and correct stacking of body parts one on top of the other. I was able to treat ballet dancers easily with my Root theory biomechanics since they have known about these mechanical flaws since 1700's.

#53 What would not be considered abnormal pronation?
1. Pronation after heel contact that is too rapid
2. Pronation after heel contact that is too prolonged
3. Pronation after heel contact excessively internally rotating the knee
4. Pronation to heel vertical in a patient with 10 degrees of tibial varum
5. Pronation to a 2 degree everted heel position before the midstance phase

(see page 139)

Signs of Excessive Supination

Common Signs of Excessive Supination
1. Lateral shift of the body weight following heel contact
2. Heel Inversion at heel contact is sometimes seen
3. No patellar internal rotation at heel contact
4. Gait sometimes appears very rigid

When you watch a person walk, the signs of excessive supination are weight transfer to the lateral side of the foot, lateral roll of the heel, lack of contact phase pronation, lack of internal rotation of the knee, loss of shock absorption or some jarring of the leg seen at heel contact, or extension of the knee at contact. There can be a slightly different presentation in every patient that calls your attention to this problem as you watch them walk. These are all clues the foot is not pronating like normal to absorb shock, and not pronating like normal to internally rotate the leg or flex the knee. Remember, contact phase pronation is crucial for normal function of the lower limb.

For some reason, unless there is a significant roll to the outside called lateral instability, many patients can not feel this motion. And, it is the motion I have the most trouble having my students in podiatry school observe correctly. In fact, in the running literature, it is often called under pronation rather than something to do with lateral motion or supination or varus positioning. It is the motion however that can be the most devastating to the body. Appendix 2 previously talked about the 20 injuries or pain locations related to this motion or position on the Supination Syndrome. It is opposite of what should happen at heel contact. Pronation of the subtalar joint is needed to absorb shock and let the entire lower extremity internally rotate smoothly until the end of the contact phase of gait. There are many muscles contracting at or just after heel contact to decelerate the pronation motion (anterior tibial, posterior tibial, gastrocnemius and soleus, flexor hallucis longus, flexor digitorum longus). If the foot is abnormally supinating, the weaker by far peroneals must do a very stressful job to try to stop supination. No wonder that they break down with the motion of abnormal supination.

#54 Which of these problems is not related to overuse of the peroneal tendons trying to decelerate abnormal heel contact supination?
1. Peroneal Tendonitis
2. Fibular Stress Fractures
3. Inversion Ankle Sprains
4. Tibial Stress Fractures
(see page 139)

When I ask a patient to walk, and it is typically in several pairs of shoes, I want them to walk at a normal pace, and sense how the weight is being distributed through their metatarsals and toes one foot at a time. I will have them focus on the right foot, and then the left, or vice versa. The two ideals, where you are not pronated or supinated at push-off, is either weight going through the first and second (never only the first) or the weight is very even to all the metatarsals. In a supinated foot at push off, you probably do not feel the first metatarsal or hallux at all. The patients really understand this when they compare feet and compare various shoes. I have found this an incredible skill to teach patients how to feel their push off, for it will help their shoe buying process their whole lives. Yet, heel contact supination typically hurts us two ways. First of all, we have heel contact supination when we should be pronating, and then secondly, we will have late midstance or early propulsive phase pronation to bring the weight back from lateral to medial. In this case, and it is the more prevalent scenario, the overall observation of the foot will be pronatory. Designing orthotic devices for this foot only for the pronation aspect will worsen the heel contact supination. When I have patients for second opinions on their orthotic devices from other physicians, this is a common reason that their current orthotic devices are not working well.

#55 As you push off through your metatarsals and toes, where is the ideal weight bearing pattern?
1. Push off through metatarsals 1 and 2
2. Push off through metatarsals 3 and 4
3. Push off through metatarsals 4 and 5
4. Push off through metatarsals 2 and 3
(see page 139)

I would rather someone pronate too much than have them supinate a little at heel contact. Any time you dispense a pair of orthotic devices, you must make sure you are not making them supinate. This is a very important observation with the Inverted Orthotic Technique, but also very important with any orthotic device or shoe selection. I was taught if my patients came back complaining of medial knee pain after getting orthotics, adjust the orthotic devices so they pronated more. Unfortunately, this can happen anytime they buy new shoes, so some good orthotic break-in advice is to always make sure they do not feel that they are rolling to the outside when they land, and at push off to make sure that they are rolling through the first and second metatarsals evenly. I tend to make my heel

cups very deep, say 21 or more mm high. This makes for a wide heel area. This can create a problem with the orthotic device not sitting down in the more narrow heel. Not only must I spot this at orthotic dispense and do some narrowing of the orthotic device to get a perfect fit, but the patient must also be aware of this when they buy other shoes and sense if the orthotic device fits properly. The patient should always try on multiple shoes to experience the difference. I explain to them that their new orthotic device will feel different in every shoe that they try on and wear. I explain that they should always feel stable and the gait smooth. There should be no pain with the process of getting used to orthotic devices.

#56 If an orthotic device forces a patient to supinate at heel contact, which one of these symptoms is typically not related?
1. Medial Knee Joint Line Pain
2. Sinus Tarsi Pain
3. Peroneal Tendon Pain
4. Sacroiliac Joint Pain
(see page 139)

One of the general rules that running stores use that is so erroneous is that flatfeet need stability or motion control shoes and high arched feet are rigid so they need cushioned shoes. There are so many problems with this general rule for all types of feet. In the high arched feet, in particular, it can be devastating. High arched feet (pes cavus) can be rigid (needing cushioned shoes), they can be laterally unstable (needing a small number of laterally stable neutral shoes like the Saucony Triumph, Brooks Ghost or Glycerin, Adidas NMD, and New Balance 1540), and they can be overpronators (needing stability or motion control shoes). The general rule fits only some of their clientele. High arched feet alone account for 10-15% of the population, and therefore 5% of all consumers that walk into a shoe store are going to be supinators on average. However, with 30% of all consumers wearing orthotic devices with the risk of becoming supinators just by wearing the wrong shoes, now 35% of all consumers could walk out of athletic shoe store in the wrong shoes causing them to supinate too much. It is our job, part of our profession, to educate stores on the problem of supination (appendix 2).

#57 With a Pes Cavus Foot Type (aka High Arches), the heel motion observed at heel contact?
1. Subtalar Joint Pronation
2. Subtalar Joint Supination
3. Subtalar Joint has No Motion
4. All of the Above
(see page 139)

Signs of Poor Shock Absorption

Common Signs of Poor Shock Absorption
1. A loud sound of heel strike
2. Shuttering of the muscles following heel contact
3. The rigid appearance of lower extremity
4. Excessive subtalar joint supination at heel contact

When you watch a patient with poor shock absorption, their legs can shutter with gait as ground reactive forces travel up the leg. You can see a fully pronated gait where there is no further pronated at heel contact, or a laterally unstable gait robbing the foot of shock absorbing pronation, but definitely not normal fluid easy contact phase pronation. It is the motion of foot pronation, leg internal rotation, with knee and hip flexion that allows us to absorb shock at heel contact or impact (in running that impact can vary positions more than walking). You may see no motion at all at the heels or the knees. You can observe a rigid trunk and upper extremity also. The lateral instability noted at heel contact, caused by the lateral shift of body weight from contact phase supination, robs the natural shock absorption from pronation. The lateral motion of the heel can be from structural deformities like tibial varum or calcaneal varus or everted forefoot deformities like plantarflexed first ray, and functional issues like peroneal tendon weakness, prior ankle sprains, shoes both new and worn that break down laterally. It is important to note that a severe pronated flatfoot may be functioning maximally pronated, so will land with tremendous shock absorption issues. It no longer has any pronation motion left to absorb shock. These feet can present with excessive jarring issues, and also abnormal positional issues where the severely pronated foot is either too everted at the heel, or too abducted to the ankle and leg.

#58 A patient with lower back pain has limb dominance noted on gait evaluation. The limb dominance may be caused by what problem?
1. Limb Length Discrepancy
2. Excessive Unilateral Pronation
3. Excessive Unilateral Supination
4. Poor Shock Absorption
5. More than one cause

(see page 139)

#59 Which deformity is typically not a cause of excessive supination?
1. Forefoot Valgus
2. Forefoot Varus
3. Tibial Varum
4. Genu Valgum
5. Prior Severe Ankle Sprains

(see page 139)

Signs of Possible Equinus

Common Signs of Equinus
1. Early Heel Off
2. Bouncy Gait with heels barely touching
3. Genu Recurvatum with excessive straightening of the knee
4. Excessive pronation typically with out-toeing gait
5. The collapse of the midfoot after heel off

As we watch someone walk, there are common presentations of tight achilles tendons. Some of the problems are typically from the chronic midfoot breakdown of the foot as the lack of bend at the ankle joint (primarily a sagittal plane force) places an abnormal and very powerful sagittal plane force on the mid foot. The rule in mechanics is that if you limit the motion at one joint, the joints above or below have to take up the stress. In ankle equinus, with a limited joint dorsiflexion, which will be primarily in the sagittal plane, the force created by the body to attempt compensation is very destructive. The two common destructive sagittal planes problems caused by equinus forces are a genu recurvatum force, which can break down the knee, or subtalar and midtarsal joint sagittal plane plantigrade collapse with pronation leading to the destruction of the midfoot and the development of a rocker bottom flat foot. It is one of the most important functions of a podiatrist to evaluate children for signs of equinus and take steps to reverse this powerful force. A standard achilles stretching problem involving the gastrocnemius, soleus, and plantar fascia gets all up and down the length of the calf muscles and the achilles tendon. The stretching should be 30 seconds in length each or 5 deep breaths. Occasionally a physical therapist or massage therapist has to be involved with deep calf mobilization of 4-8 sessions. When there is the stubborn case of tightness that needs a prolonged heat then ice routine that will be described in Appendix 7.

Early Heel Off
As just alluded to, a sagittal plane deformity such as tight Achilles' tendons compensates mainly in the sagittal plane

. Drs. Root and Weed professed this general rule in helping students and surgeons understand what forces could be controlled with orthotic devices and which couldn't be controlled and needed other forms of treatment. Early heel off, meaning that heel lift occurs closer to the middle of midstance when our bodies are still over our ankles and not in front of the ankles. This is when the ankles are not bent into the 10 degrees of dorsiflexion that is normal and can be transiently associated with growth spurts where the bones are growing faster than the tendons in children. It can also occur at any time in life we let our achilles get too tight. It is so important to carefully measure the Achilles flexibility with the gold standard being ankle joint dorsiflexion with the subtalar neutral as described in Appendix 5. This was established since in normal stance, heel lift should occur there should be a ten degree ankle dorsiflexed position when the subtalar joint is close to neutral (typically within a few degrees). This examination technique has great reliability for the examiner. If you see any of the signs of equinus, yet do not measure equinus, it is important to work with your colleagues or teachers to see what your test error is. The most common error is typically allowing the subtalar joint to pronate while dorsiflexing the ankle, which can give you 10-15 degrees more. Of course, the early heel lift can be totally neurological (hyperinnervation of the calf muscles) and have nothing to do with achilles tightness.

Bouncy Gait

This is an extension of early heel off where the heels typically do not spend much time, if at all, on the ground. As in all equinus conditions, this can be seen in growth spurts. Bouncy gaits are also seen in hyperactive nervous systems a little more than early heel off patients. Many of my bouncy gait patients have no equinus at all. Thus, we have to measure the flexibility to see what we are dealing with so appropriate treatment can be started. The patterns of early heel off and bouncy gait are not as serious if there is no equinus associated with it. They both overload the metatarsals which can develop pain. Toe runners, with or without equinus, can have a bouncy gait.

Genu Recurvatum

Here is where the ability to recognize and appropriately rehabilitate equinus can prevent the long term breakdown of knee joints. The force of genu recurvatum is produced by a tight gastrocnemius which crosses the knee joint axis originating on the back of the femur. The tight musculature pulls the femur posteriorly and inferiorly on the tibia. The knee is seen to buckle somewhat posteriorly or hyperextend when it should be flexing in contact and the early part of midstance. To some observers the knee just looks too straight, and that loss of knee flexion following heel contact means that the knee joint will look stiff. This is such a strong force that even the treatment has difficulties. If you ask these patients to stretch the gastrocnemius with the knee straight, the knee may hyper-extend in the process, making things worse. This patient must keep the knee joint ever so slightly bent while stretching, somewhat taking a slower course. If you suspect this condition, it is good to have the patient in tight pants or shorts when measuring. As you dorsiflex the ankle, carefully watch the knee joint and stop the measurement at any signs of recurvatum force at the knee joint. The patient actually hyperextends the knee during the measuring process to attempt to gain more ankle dorsiflexion.

Out Toe Gait

This is an example of a sagittal plane force compensating in the transverse plane. Typically in general compensation for any problem occurs in the easiest way possible. So, patients with very strong and tight achilles compensate with bounce to some degree. Patients with some out toe anyway can compensate by simply toeing out further. But what does this out toeing actually do? If you lack normal ankle joint dorsiflexion, by externally rotating the foot, you can use subtalar joint pronation instead of ankle joint dorsiflexion to move forward. Dr. Root emphasized that frontal plane forces were the easiest to treat, sagittal plane second, and transverse plane the hardest. By recognizing that the out toeing was a transverse plane compensation, your treatment success of the equinus condition and the overall biomechanics will be easier.

Late Midstance to Propulsive Arch Collapse

As the patient walks, they move from heel contact, into midstance, and then push off the ground. With equinus, as the patient gets to midstance the tibia can not bend forward due to the stiff ankle, so the subtalar joint stays pronated keeping the midtarsal

joint loose. This laxity of the midtarsal joint allows the arch to collapse along with first ray dorsiflexion easily helping the body to move forward over a pronated foot. It is subtalar joint prolonged pronation, midtarsal joint oblique axis pronation, first ray dorsiflexion, and midtarsal joint longitudinal axis supination that gets this done. All of these abnormal motions or positions can be devastating to the foot with bunions, hallux limitus, hammertoes, neuromas, plantar fasciitis, etc developing (see Appendix 1 and the foot pronatory symptoms).

#60 Equinus is such a powerful force on the body and lower extremity that the gait signs are numerous and damaging. Which one of the following is a common equinus sign?
1. Outtoe Gait
2. Early Heel Lift
3. Excessive Pronation
4. Midfoot arch collapse
5. Bouncy Gait
6. Apropulsive Gait
7. Genu Recurvatum
8. All of the above

(see page 139)

Signs of Weak Muscles

Common Signs of Typical Severely Weak Muscles
1. Medial arch collapse with weak posterior tibial tendon
2. Lack of heel lift with weak achilles complex
3. Excessive internal patellar rotation with weak external hip rotators

4. Lean to one side with weak hip abductors
5. Contact Phase Lateral Instability with weak peroneal tendons

As you watch someone perform an activity, there are normal motions which demonstrate proper technique or form for that activity. This applies to the basic activities of walking and running, but also ballet, cycling, rowing, bench pressing, etc. As you observe these activities, weak muscles can present as a subtle or a very gross problem. Most subtleties are picked up on muscle testing and grading of muscles. We all know when patients present with knee pain that we have to test quadriceps and hamstring strength, but maybe the real problem is more subtle in gluteus medius or posterior tibial or soleus weaknesses. So, there are subtleties even in manual testing. Gait evaluation only suggests weaknesses by the pattern of motion seen. After observing various patterns of motion, it can be fun to see if there are weak muscles involved. So often with our athletes, the examination really should be done after an athlete fatigues the muscle in physical activity, but that may not be practical in the office setting. If my examination does not match the suspected physical examination findings, I often ask my patients to workout for at least an hour just before their next examination if that is at all possible. Let us discuss the signs of weak muscles above one by one.

The Collapsed Arch
As we watch a patient walk, we notice medial arch collapse on one or both sides.

Of course, as with all motions, it may be caused by a single muscle weakness, a whole group of weak muscles, or have nothing to do with a weak muscle (for example, torn spring ligament or forefoot varus deformity and its compensation). But, we know that this finding of an excessively collapsed arch is a problem that is not part of the normal technique of walking, and we want to investigate the problem further. Appendix 1 explained all the places pain can develop with overpronation, so this same patient may be presenting with 2-3 or more problems that they felt unrelated to the collapsed arch. These problems may be in their feet, ankles, shins, knees, hips and low back. Yet, all or part of these pain patterns may have developed with this over pronation and will improve with over pronation treatments. I had a patient recently that 15 of her 17 lower extremity complaints were helped after good orthotic devices was made. She knew she pronated and that caused arch pain, and some ankle symptoms, but she did not realize most of the rest of her complaints (knees, hips, back, and neck) were also related. It was not until she received a fairly corrective orthotic device that more and more of her symptoms began to disappear.

In the above patient, the arch collapse was severe and caused by a very weak posterior tibial tendon (PTTD Stage 2). Sometimes, it is the anterior tibial tendon that can be a problem, or part of the problem also. The Achilles complex has a strong medial attachment in the heel to help decelerate contact phase pronation and cause heel supination at heel lift, so weakness there can also cause pronation with destabilization of the medial column. Treatment cannot just support the collapsed stressed tissue, but also a very thorough and thoughtful strengthening program. Taping and orthotic devices may be a temporary or permanent aspect of the treatment, but they are definitely needed until the tissue gets stronger. With the barefoot controversy came a clearer understanding that orthotic devices for some problems are necessary casts needed only in the Immobilization Phase of an injury, some are needed only throughout the 3 Phases of Rehabilitation, and some more permanently at least in high stress activities. If a patient can get by with limited or no overall disability, I would not recommend surgery for the collapsed foot. It is the cases I see of adult acquired flat feet that may need surgery so I co-treat these patients with a surgeon who I trust can perform such surgery.

Poor Heel Lift

As your body moves through gait, at the end of midstance, your heel should lift off the ground as the body weight is transferred forward. In propulsion, after heel lift, the body weight get smoothly transferred to the other foot that is beginning the contact phase. When that heel lift does not occur, the patient shuffles forward, the gait is called apropulsive. This is a very damaging gait. There is excessive weight on the heels and forefoot, the hips must lift the feet off the ground with excessive hip flexion called steppage gait. The knees are stiff in mid stance as the weight is held back. It is hard to miss this gait. The history typically from the patient is damaged low back with neurological defect, or someone with very weak Achilles' tendon or tendons from old injuries with and without surgery. The ability to do a single heel raise is not only vital to normal gait, it is vital to all weight bearing activities, and should be part of our examination when poor heel lift is detected.

Excessive Internal Patellar Rotation

The "squinting patella" is produced by excessive internal rotation of the femur at the contact phase of gait. It actually can be only seen on one side, or both. It may be observed in walking and running, or just with the higher forces observed in running. As you land on the ground, your lower limb is internally rotating. The internal rotation can be excessive in amount, speed, or duration. Of course, an excessively internal patella can be purely structural caused by internal femoral torsion. The typical biomechanical examination measures the internal and external rotation of the hip which should be quite equal and points to structural issues if more internal or external is noted in this passive examination. Then the muscle strength and flexibility of the internal and external rotators is evaluated. Two common findings are found: weak external rotators alone, or weak internal and external rotators combined. Either way, after you strike the ground, the normal internal rotation of the femur must be decelerated by the external hip rotators. If they are weak, the internal rotation can be too much, prolonged, too rapid, or the end point of the knee positioned too far out of alignment (not stacked up correctly). The patella appears to be cross eyed or squinting.

Dominance to One Side (Side Lean)

When you watch a patient walk down the hallway, I love to have them do this activity multiple times to look for patterns. If you see a slight shift to one side whether they are walking towards you or away from you, it could mean that they have a short leg syndrome. The general rule, which has many exceptions, is that we fall (dominant) to our longer side. This is by far the most common cause of limb dominance. A less common cause of this side lean is weak hip abductors. As the patient loads the weight bearing foot, if the hip abductors are weak, the body falls or leans to the opposite non weight bearing side "trendelenburg gait". This is opposite in cases where there is trunk instability and the body shifts over the supporting hip to seek stability. And, of course, it can be purely caused by limping or favoring, where the patient leans away from pain (as in hip arthritis). Therefore, if you are watching a patient that can not stay centered, or stacked up correctly, as they walk and lean to one side, check for weak abductors, short leg syndrome, limited hip range of motion, and also a good history of their hip, pelvis, and low back pain. You may be the one that helps someone decide on hip replacement, low back evaluation, physical therapy evaluation, and of course, the appropriate MD consult. I recently treated a patient with hip pain on the side they collapsed towards. Cortisone shot for a hip bursitis was not helpful. Three different opinions came up with 3 sources of pain: low back, hip itself, and referred pain from the knee. A ¾ inch leg length was found and treated and all the symptoms disappeared. The already scheduled hip replacement was indefinitely cancelled.

Contact Phase Lateral Instability

Excessive supination, also called under pronation, or lateral instability should not occur after heel contact. The foot should be pronating with the internally rotating lower limb in the contact phase. This foot pronation makes the foot looser and more adaptable to the irregular ground. This foot pronation also allows us to absorb shock along with contact phase knee and hip flexion. I have always said I would rather a patient pronate a lot than supinate at the wrong time a little. As you supinate, and the weight bearing shifts laterally, the peroneal tendons (longus, brevis, and somewhat tertius) attempt to stabilize the lateral side of the foot and ankle. If these tendons are weak in general, or never re-strengthened after an ankle sprain, they can not protect the lateral ankle and more inversion can occur. It may be a young gal who has normal mechanics, but the peroneal tendons are so weak that she can not wear high heels or ice skate. A good strengthening program for the peroneal tendons can completely stabilize the ankle in 80% of patients. The 20% may need orthotics, high tops, braces, taping, and/or surgical treatments.

#61 As we watch gait, there are many signs that our muscles are not performing well.

Match the following weak muscles to the gait finding.

1. Posterior Tibial Weakness
2. External Hip Rotator Weakness
3. Achilles/Calf Weakness
4. Hip Abductor Weakness
5. Peroneal Weakness

Gait Finding:

1. Lateral Ankle Instability
2. Excessive Hip Lean (Side Dominance)
3. Excessive Pronation
4. Excessive Internal Femoral Rotation
5. Absence of Heel Lift

(see page 139)

Examples of Gait Findings and Treatment Options

Example #1

A runner presents after developing left knee pain on a long training run preparing for the San Francisco Marathon that is in two months. Gait evaluation revealed a dominance (or body shift) to the left side suggesting at least more weight bearing on the injured left side and perhaps a short leg syndrome. This dominance to the injured side is also significant due to the fact it is the opposite of mere favoring to take the load off the injury. The left knee had a more internal rotation at heel contact on the side of the runner's knee complaint. The heel was actually inverting at heel contact (opposite force of knee internal rotation). The patient was then asked to run up and down along hallway with the running shoes that they brought into the office. It was a brand new pair, as they had purchased them in hopes it would clear up the knee problem.

I asked the patient to bring in the pair she was wearing when she hurt the knee to the next visit.

Remember the Rule of 3 in evaluating these overuse injuries. Any injury, where the tissue is so overstressed that it begins to complain, typically has at least 3 causes. This is why one patient with overuse, or overpronation, or wears inadequate shoes, can develop knee pain, another shin splints, another foot pain, and so on. It is a fun investigation which, of course, should be started on the first visit on the new problem or new injury. In this case, the left knee was being stressed by:

1. An inadequate training base and overall program (she was up to 15 miles only two months after starting running)
2. A dominance to the left probably placing 20% or more weight on the left side (later found that is was the long leg of a ¼ inch)
3. Excessive internal patellar rotation caused by very weak hip external rotators (quickly improved with an appropriate strengthening program)
4. Unstable athletic shoes with poor support causing excessive contact phase supination and cushion (discovered at the second visit)
5. Other components discovered in subsequent visits were weak quadriceps, tight hamstrings, and low Vitamin D (not sure if there was a relationship here)

So, gait evaluation pointed the way to several key components that were easy to correct in the long run (no pun intended). This particular patient would go on to run several marathons over the next few years with strong external hip rotators and quads, a good and safer training program, Brooks Glycerin Shoes for her supination, and a Sole OTC insert that I could place a slight valgus wedge also for the supination . She knows she has one leg longer, and someday that may need to be addressed. She reversed the Vitamin D deficiency, and if she breaks anything a bone density will be ordered. Her primary care physician thought that at 32 years old, and no history of fractures, a bone density scan was not called for in this case. It took 6 months to get the external hip rotators strong, and initially, the therapist was not isolating the external hip rotators enough and not stretching the tight upper part of the medial hamstrings. When you imagine that the average beginning runner quits running within a year of starting, runners really appreciate this type of approach towards wellness and long-term prevention. This example also points out that you do not need to always correct everything at once.

Example #2

This 76 year old noticed pain in the lateral side of her left foot 6 months before her appointment that had been getting worse and more limiting. She also noted some flattening of her left foot in the last few months. Gait evaluation showed markedly more pronation on the left foot compared to the uninvolved right foot, with heel valgus only seen on the left side. She noted swelling medially, but the pain was only lateral. We are obviously dealing with posterior tibial tendon dysfunction but it is not the usual location of pain. By again using our Rule of 3, the examination found (more than 3 for sure):

1. Very weak posterior tibial tendon
2. Very weak Achilles' tendon with overstretched length
3. 12-degree heel valgus resting position measured on the left side, and 3 degrees valgus or everted heel position on the right side.
4. The tendency to always wear heels or flats with no support
5. 30-year-old left ankle sprain with questionable rehabilitation
6. Not an ounce of athletic sense or body awareness in our conversations or her task performances
7. Overweight
8. Inactive her whole life (busy professional until retirement at 71 years old)

Gait evaluation pointed to the pronation problem left greater than right. The significant heel valgus would have been missed without gait analysis. She had been dealing with weak muscles for a long time, but the heel valgus was causing lateral ankle impingement. MRI showed some irregularities in the posterior tibial tendon but no tear. She really had pronation pain, not posterior tibial tendon dysfunction pain. She knew she had neglected her health, but fought diligently to take stress off the lateral ankle and was quite simple to treat in some ways. The 6 things that turned her symptoms around:

1. Stable shoes and ⅜ th inch varus wedge (¼ inch for the uninvolved right side)
2. Joined Weight Watchers and lost 22 in 3 months
3. Began a one year program of posterior tibial, Achilles, single leg balancing, external hip rotator strengthening (probably had doubled her initial strength in the first 2 months)
4. Icing 3 times daily for anti-inflammatory
5. Leukotape with coverall to prevent heel eversion (helped the varus wedge)
   https://youtu.be/AcSSyBfFocE
6. Several dressier flats that could not hold the internal varus wedge had ¼ inch varus outsole wedging applied full length by a local cobbler.

I am not mentioning the functional orthotics she received in the things that turned her around because she was so much better months before they were dispensed, and I actually never saw her wear them except at the orthotic dispense visit 4 months into our journey together. She was given highly corrective orthotic devices for the left (35 degrees), and 20 degrees for the lesser pronated right foot. Both athletic and dress versions were made, and because Medicare does not pay for them, she self-paid for this and only this part of the treatments. She said they were in some hiking boots, but she always came into the visits in dress shoes with the outsole varus wedge. The shoes she brought into the dispense visit could not fit either pair, so I actually never saw her wear them.

I said that she was easy to treat in some ways because the real reason I remember her is that the first podiatrist she saw immediately used the "S" word. This podiatrist did watch her walk, and saw the pronation. She was immediately placed into the adult acquired flat foot reconstruction category, and without MRI or a lot of thought, had scheduled her for flat foot reconstruction with the breaking of the heel bone, fusion of some joint, and repairing of tendons. She only saw me because a friend had seen me and told her at least just to get another opinion. I only saw her five times, about one month apart. The first visit was an hour and we talked about the surgery for 45 minutes of the visit. The next visits were 30 minutes each and each visit we talked about the surgery a little less and less. The last visit, when she was completely out of pain, walking 30 minutes daily, there was no discussion of surgery until as she left the office she turned around and said: "how will I know when I need surgery?" The power of a word. I saw her one year later for follow up and an ingrown toenail, she looked 20 years younger, 37 lb weight loss overall, exercising regularly and did not say the "S" word at all.

#62 Gait Evaluation is crucial to the treatment of many lower extremity problems. Proper gait evaluation should be with new and old broken down shoes. If the patient is an athlete, gait evaluation should include running because you can run very differently than you walk. Which of the following rule does not apply to gait evaluation?

1. You should always watch a runner run on the first visit since it can affect treatment
2. Patients when calling for their first appointment should be told to bring the shoes they normally wear
3. Patients should be told to bring in a running or athletic shoe with the most wear
4. No treatment decisions about shoe gear and orthotic devices should be done when the patient is limping, or can not run or walk.

(see page 139)

#63 An abnormal motion like excessive rearfoot pronation affects the weakest link in the chain. This can be in the foot, ankle, leg, knee, hip or low back. Why an area is weak in the first place is multifactorial. Which of the following is not typically why the posterior tibial insertional area gets sore?

1. Over pronation
2. Weak Posterior Tibial Tendon
3. Metatarsus Primus Elevatus
4. Weak Peroneus Brevis Tendon
5. Weak Achilles Tendon
6. Os Tibial Externum Presence

(see page 139)

Appendix 5: Basic Components of a Lower Extremity Biomechanical Examination

There are many basic examination components to a Lower Extremity Biomechanical Examination. The "Biomechanical Exam" that I utilize is summarized here and I will emphasize the importance of each part. Various teachers of the biomechanical examination may and will have their own version. Every student should learn all the aspects of a good biomechanical examination, and practitioners use the aspects of this examination that apply to each individual patient. I love to make observations walking first, then standing, and finally laying (prone then supine). The Gait Evaluation Checklist in Appendix 4 is more thorough and can replace the gait findings part of the biomechanical examination.

Patient's Name_____
Date_____

Gait Findings:

Plane of Deformity
(Right) Sagittal_____
(Left) Sagittal_____
(Right) Transverse_____
(Left) Transverse_____
(Right) Frontal_____
(Left) Frontal_____

Hip/Knee Transverse and Frontal Plane Issues
(Right)_____
(Left)_____

Summary of Gait Findings
(Right)_____
_____
_____
_____
_____
(Left)_____
_____
_____
_____
_____

Standing Findings:

LLD Landmarks
IC Higher_____
ASIS Higher _____
GT Higher _____
PSIS Higher_____

Overall Structure
(Right)_____
_____
(Left)_____
_____

RCSP
(Right)_____
(Left)_____

NCSP
(Right)_____
(Left)_____

Neutral Tibial Position

(Right)_____

(Left)_____

Functional Hallux Limitus (barefoot alone)
Right _____ Left_____
With Orthosis
Right_____ Left_____

Hubscher Maneuver (and Jack's Test)
(Right)_____
(Left)_____

Single Leg Heel Raise
(Right)_____
(Left)_____

Single Leg Balance
(Right)_____
(Left)_____

Patient Lying Prone:

AJDF
(Right) straight_____ bent_____
(Left)   straight_____ bent_____

Forefoot Deformity
(Right)_____ (Left)_____
After mobilization (if varus)
(Right)_____ (Left) _____

First Ray Range of Motion
Right (Up)_____ (Down)_____
Left (Up)_____ (Down)_____

STJ NP
(Right) Inv___ Ev___ NP___
(Left) Inv____ Ev____ NP___

Patient Lying Supine:

Subtalar Joint Axis
Right_____
Left_____
MTJ ROM
(Right)_____
(Left)_____

Further Strength Testing
(Right) Inversion_____
(Left) Inversion_____
(Right) Eversion_____
(Left) Eversion_____
(Right) Dorsiflexion_____
(Left) Dorsiflexion_____

This represents my basic biomechanical evaluation to get a sense of the forces that are causing an injury and need to be reversed (those that I can treat in some way). These are not all of my biomechanical assessment tools, as they should not be for you. The following list are other common evaluations that are done sporatically based on the patient's problems:

1. Hip Range of Motion (hip pain problems or getting an overall assessment of internal and external issues)
2. Malleolar Torsion (overall assessment of internal and external problems)

3. Angle of Gait (overall assessment of internal and external problems and resultant pronation or supination issues)
4. Quad and Hamstring Strength and Flexibility (knee pain problems or getting overall assessment of gait findings or equinus forces)
5. Metatarsal Arch (overall assessment of each ray positioning for metatarsal issues)
6. Other muscle strength tests appropriate for the injury or gait findings.

I think each professor in biomechanics is okay to have their own versions. This is a modified version of what I learned 43 years ago. The basics for both the student and practitioner to learn from your examination is:

1. How stable is this patient?
2. How easy will it be for me to make them more stable?
3. How strong is this patient?
4. How does what I find structurally compare to what I find in gait?

There are many components to the foot evaluation that are utilized by a biomechanical specialist in assessing their patients and determining treatment plans. These examinations are the crucial findings in a full mechanical evaluation. Some podiatrists always perform every examination in a certain order called "the biomechanical examination". It is crucial that some order like this happens in the podiatric medical schools, or in biomechanical workshops at seminars, for practice is needed to get a feel for these tests and what they mean. In the real life of clinical practice, some podiatrists tend to be selective in what they measure based on what they think is important for an individual patient. Like Mulder testing is important only when you think a Morton's Neuroma or plantar plate tear may be present, and Thompson testing is important only when you are testing for a suspected Achilles rupture, there are certain biomechanical tests that are important for metatarsal patients, Achilles tendinitis patients, etc. I like to perform my historical review, then watch the patient walk and/or run, and measure on that visit what I think is crucial. What do I need to know now? I hope as I discuss the common biomechanical examinations of the foot and lower extremity I will give you some indication why they are needed and measured. You are trying to categorize the patient in your initial visit to come up with Plan A (with other plans down the line since we have to start somewhere).

I want to briefly comment on the importance of performing these tests. In reality, there are going to be differences in how you and I exactly measure the individual angles. However, you are going to see the bell shaped curve of each deformity just the same as I will, and that will give you a sense of when to treat or not treat. If you look at the next one hundred patients doing each test, you will easily get a sense of which patients are tight and which are loose, or which patients are pronated and which are supinated, or which have a tight midtarsal joint and which have ligamentous laxity. These findings may be very important for your understanding of the patient's mechanics and how you eventually treat them. Your whole practice of Podiatry could delve into the depths of these examinations and their treatments. To understand the Inverted Orthotic Technique well, you need some knowledge of these tests to decipher what the patient is telling you, and how they are responding to the changes you are making.

Let's look at a very common example of someone that may walk into your office on a daily basis. They present with leg pain above the inside of the ankle from running. The pain came on gradually over the last several months and now they can not run more than several miles without the pain worsening. They have had no treatment except some store bought arch supports and a change in shoes after the store noticed that they had high arches. Upon questioning, there has been no swelling, and no pain with walking. Only running bothers them. There are no nerve like symptoms. There is definitely an overuse aspect because they had increased their daily mileage and have been running 6 days a week (poor recovery times). Prior problems were plantar fasciitis and runner's medial knee symptoms. As a podiatrist, you are categorizing these under excessive pronation injuries (see appendix 1), although the pes cavus foot type may tend to supinate more than pronate. You then watch the patient walk and they have contact phase pronation, not the expected supination. You watch the person run, and pronation is severe. It is common to have different biomechanics walking and running. Luckily, you have trained your front desk to

tell all the patients with sports injuries to bring shorts and old and new shoes for the visit. Because of the high arch, the last pair recommended by the running store using general rules (pes cavus gets neutral shoes) were neutral shoes for cushion which made the pronation worse. The pair of shoes that the injury began was light stability and pronation was still significantly more on the injured side. Your physical examination is to identify the structure injured, and get an idea of the biomechanics. This is another example of asymmetrical function which will need asymmetrical treatment (definitely higher support on the more pronated side). At another visit, you may have them schedule for the complete biomechanical examination. Why does this pes cavus foot pronate? You find that the posterior tibial tendon is sore on palpation and contraction against resistance, and it is also extremely weak (muscle strength is an important aspect of the biomechanics of any patient). You find the pronation may be driven by very tight achilles tendons which you measure, document, and can check if the patient's stretching regimen is helping in future visits. You find a tibial varum causing pronation to vertical only, so varus wedging or canting is needed. You find a hypermobile first ray (over 20 mm of first ray motion) so as the first metatarsal head tries to take weight it dorsiflexes too much leaving the medial column unstable. The examinations that helped you decide on future treatments were: muscle testing, equinus testing, first ray range of motion, relaxed and neutral calcaneal positions, and of course gait evaluation especially of running for a runner.

In appendix 4 the gait evaluation was focused on the common findings that patients present with to your office. The patient you are treating most likely had some findings. Your job is to ascertain if the findings have anything to do with their symptoms, and if you can help change the biomechanics for the better. Before we look at the examination tests, let's discuss what we are looking for in these tests. It is fun to start with syndromes which have been previously discussed: pronation syndrome (appendix 1), supination syndrome (appendix 2), etc. Here are some of the possible reasons you think that they have developed their symptoms which can be applied to every initial patient until you begin to categorize them:

- Excessive pronation caused the symptoms
- Excessive supination caused the symptoms
- Limb Length Difference caused the symptoms
- Poor Shock Absorption caused the symptoms
- Tight Tendons caused the symptoms
- Weak Muscles caused the symptoms
- Various Instabilities caused the symptoms

How then do we evaluate for these? How do we evaluate for excessive pronation? How do we evaluate for excessive supination? How do we evaluate for all the mechanical causes of injury? This is the important role of gait evaluation teamed up with the biomechanical examination. We initially develop a Plan A, and should be thinking of B and C maybe?

There are so many subtleties to the art of medicine and the field of biomechanics is part of it. Podiatrists, such as I, can spend their whole careers trying to find out why someone hurts and how to fix it. Other podiatrists might be involved with the Acute Phase, and refer to physical therapists for the rehabilitation. Some podiatrists are involved solely with the rehabilitation without much biomechanical knowledge, but I love to figure out the why's that a biomechanical approach can help immensely, which gets you into the entire rehabilitative process. Is it a dropped metatarsal, too much pronation or supination, a leg length difference, tight or weak muscles, or too much shock going up their legs. As we get into the common biomechanical examinations, remember that the more tests you learn, the more you will understand how they apply to your patients.

Gait Findings:

Plane of Deformity Evaluation

Plane of Deformity (check what you observe as the number one force for each side)

(Right) Sagittal_____
(Left) Sagittal_____
(Right) Transverse_____
(Left) Transverse_____
(Right) Frontal_____
(Left) Frontal_____

This was one of the most memorable rules for me from Dr. Root. When you are assessing a patient's biomechanics, you will find which plane of deformity stands out the most. Is the primary plane of deformity frontal, sagittal, or transverse? In terms of custom orthotic corrections, Dr. Root's rule was that frontal plane deformities are the easiest to treat, then sagittal plane, with transverse plane the hardest to correct. Even though when you stabilize the tri-plane motion of the foot with orthotic devices, you still stabilize the frontal plane the most as you correct for varus or valgus conditions. I have used this rule my whole career relying on the Inverted Technique for better transverse plane stability, along with other treatments that will effect that plane (like strengthening hip external rotators when there is too much internal rotation). Sagittal plane deformities are limb length discrepancies, tight Achilles' tendons, and tight hamstrings which can put tremendous force on the foot collapsing the arch. The collapse of the arch can be caused by sagittal deformities, and protected by custom orthotic devices to some degree, but the treatment has to be directed at the cause ultimately (lifts for short legs and stretching for tight muscles). Pronation, when produced by transverse and sagittal plane deformities and the forces that they create, should be treated by the Inverted Technique along with the appropriate ancillary treatments of lifts, shoes, strength, flexibility, activity modifications, etc.

#64 Which of the following transverse plane deformities may produce excessive subtalar joint pronation especially in the transverse plane requiring the Inverted Orthotic Technique?

1. Internal Femoral Torsion
2. External Femoral Torsion
3. Internal Malleolar Torsion
4. External Malleolar Torsion
5. High Subtalar Joint Axis
6. Metatarsus Adductus
7. All of the Above

(see page 139)

Dr. Root discovered that the most damaging aspect of pronation was on the subluxation side of the joint. So, if you pronate past the end range of motion of a joint, this is when it is the most damaging and most painful. Think about the midfoot collapse created by tight achilles. The tight achilles is producing a sagittal plane pronatory subluxation force across the midfoot. A rocker bottom foot is created primarily in the sagittal plane by this sagittal plane force. This is also the reason when you use corrective or highly corrective orthoses like the Inverted Orthotic Technique, you must try to eliminate the subluxation pronation forces produced by equinus, limb length discrepancies, and transverse plane problems.

#65 A patient is prescribed Inverted Orthotic Devices since they pronate too much. The prescription was based on relaxed calcaneal stance position only without ever developing an understanding of why the patient pronated in the first place. What would be the order of simplest to hardest pronation forces to control? List in the answer sheet on page 139.

1. Forefoot Varus 7 Degrees
2. Tight Achilles Tendons producing pronation
3. External Femoral Torsion producing pronation

(see page 139)

Every podiatrist in practice has made a great pair of custom made functional foot orthoses, correcting the foot mechanics close to perfect, only to find out the patient had too much arch pain. So, you need to temporarily adjust the arch to make it more comfortable (Step 1), but now in this compromised biomechanical state you need to find out what forces you are dealing with that allow the foot to pronate on the device causing pain and discomfort (Step 2). You could just attempt to undercorrect the arch by switching to a Modified Root and Medial Kirby Skive, or Inverted Orthotic Technique (possibly Step 3). But, it is best, if you felt the correction was initially perfect, to delve into the biomechanical examination and look for pronatory forces that can be corrected (better Step 3). Here is a partial list of these forces that are commonly in play in my practice (some of these forces may require surgery to correct completely):

1. Internal or External Hip Deformities helped by strengthening and gait changes
2. Limb Length Discrepancies helped by lifts under the short leg
3. Tight Achilles and hamstrings needing stretching, and at times PT and braces (like the new DeHeer Equinus Brace).
4. Internal or External Tibial or Malleolar Torsion helped by gait changes, gait plates, and some strengthening
5. High Subtalar Joint Axis or Loose Midtarsal Joint or Metatarsus Adductus causing forefoot abduction on the rearfoot (needing wide shoes to accommodate and a daily progressive foot strengthening).

Hip/Knee Transverse and Frontal Plane Issues

Hip/Knee Transverse and Frontal Plane Issues
(Right)_____
(Left)_____

As you watch gait, the position of the knee is the best to observe where the hip joint is functioning: relatively straight, excessively external, or excessively internal. It is the internal and external that may need the Inverted Orthotic Technique the most, but even the frontal plane deformity of excessive genu valgum can be helped by the varus heel positioning helped with the Inverted Orthotic Technique. There are exceptions to every rule and some patients with genu valgum compensate by excessive supination at the rearfoot. This will be so obvious in gait and no consideration of an Inverted Orthotic Device would be considered. Genu varus deformities typically need valgus foot corrections. This was another of Dr. Root's rules: standard functional foot orthotic devices are best for intrinsic foot deformities over extrinsic forces from above the foot. Dr. Root came to understand that the Inverted Orthotic Technique has more power to potentially help if the pronatory force was coming from above the foot like genu valgum, internal femoral rotation, or external femoral rotation.

#66 Excessive foot pronation which can cause one or many symptoms (see appendix 1) may be easy to treat or hard to treat. When the force of pronation is severe, and the problem/injury above the foot, the Inverted Orthotic Technique gives you the most power to correct this pronatory force. Besides the actual foot orthotic device, what are other needed treatments to help control pronation?
1. Strengthening Externally Rotating Muscles
2. Stretching equinus producing Tendons
3. Correcting for Limb Length Discrepancies (typically pronating one limb more than the other)
4. Changing Workouts to lessen stress overall by varying workouts, changing recovery times, cross training, etc.
5. Gait Training modifications (less rearfoot pronation typically when changing strike patterns)
6. All of the above (it is usually a slow progressive program)

Summary of Gait Findings

Summary of Gait Findings:

(Right)_____
_____
_____
_____
(Left)_____
_____
_____
_____

For many complicated patients, I actually use my own gait evaluation form or checklist from Appendix 4. But, for our purposes here for the standard situation, a simple summary of all of the striking or most notable findings can be noted here. You are typically categorizing patients as pronators, supinators, signs of leg length, tight or weak muscles and poor shock absorption. Other striking abnormalities like postural sway, poor hip motion, forefoot strike patterns, or varus knee jerk may be memorable and someday help with your examinations and treatments. It is important to note asymmetries or differences between the two sides. As you treat, you typically want to see that asymmetry smooth out if not reversed. Keep focus on both this asymmetry and the primary plane of deformity (if it is obvious). Most prescriptions for the Inverted Technique should capture that asymmetry. Many patients that you are debating to use Root vs Inverted will be swayed towards Inverted by that mere fact that the pronation is driven by forces above the foot and that these pronatory forces are primarily transverse or sagittal plane forces.

Standing Findings:

Now that we have looked at gait, and have drawn some conclusions on the presenting biomechanics, I have the patient stop in front of me to look at their limb length landmarks first and then move down towards the foot.

Limb Length Discrepancy Landmarks

LLD Landmarks
IC Higher_____
ASIS Higher _____
GT Higher _____
PSIS Higher_____

Statistically 80% of patients have a structural leg length difference, and almost everyone functions asymmetrically due to variations from right side to left side in muscle power, right or left handed dominance, old injuries, flexibility, and other structural or functional differences. Asymmetry is the rule not the exception. If you have done gait evaluation first, you should be able to easily spot differences, which may end up helping the treatment. You are simply an educated observer here making observations. With 80% of all adults over 60 with back pain of some sort, the treatment of leg length differences should be more widespread. I have found as little as a 1/16th of an inch can make a big difference in a world class cyclist or rower trying to avoid tissue stress in repetitive motions, and ⅛ to ⅜ inch helpful in more normal activity patients. It is my go-to treatment for back and hip issues. Being a podiatrist, I treat the part I can, and putting things like lifts in shoes is my forte. Having done this for so many years, and treating patients that are seeing some of the smartest minds in medicine, I can honestly say to my podiatry students that their contribution for that patient with knee, hip and back pain may be the most important. Like anything, when a hundred patients have the same problem, and if you could guarantee that they all got the same treatment, they would fall into camps of what was the most important aspect to their treatment. Using lift therapy for short leg syndrome will give you some patients that can not tolerate them (on one side of the spectrum) to some patients that it is the most important part (on the other side of the spectrum).

The landmarks for leg length evaluation are:
1. Anterior superior iliac spines
2. Posterior superior iliac spines
3. Iliac crests
4. Greater Trochanter

These are typically done barefoot with the knees straight, or with orthotics if you are happy with the correction and no orthotic changes are anticipated. Your hands should be parallel with the floor and your eyes at the level you are trying to observe. I always ask the patient if they feel I am on the same spot right to left, and occasionally they have to advise me to raise or lower one hand.

One thing to remember, even though pretty accurate, and far better than using tape measures, it is not accurate more than 80% of patients. Measuring, and then treating, structural limb length discrepancies is then very important when you believe that the injury or pain pattern is related. After you put lifts in the shoe, you should then observe an improvement in gait. I treat the podiatric part of low back pain with some physiatrists and other medical doctors. I have seen so many great successes with chronic back pain and leg length differences. Lifts for short leg typically remove the sagittal plane force of pronation. This is not the force producing forefoot abduction on the rearfoot (transverse plane), it is the force that flattens the arch driving the foot onto the orthotic device making it uncomfortable and forcing you to adjust (sagittal plane). I love to keep my lifts full length (to the sulcus) so it lifts the heel and ball of the foot together. I also love to keep my lifts separate from the orthotic devices as you try to make things comfortable, and figure out the role of each treatment modality.

#67 The use of heel lifts in the treatment for short legs is the standard in the industry. However, heel lifts should be changed to sulcus length or full length lifts at times due to:
1. Runners who spend much of their time on the ball of the foot
2. Patients who are already unstable in their ankles and need more than ⅛ inch lift
3. Patients who are complaining about arch, shin or knee pain after heel lifts are initiated
4. All of the above
(see page 139)

Overall Structure

Overall Structure
(Right)_____
_____
_____
(Left)_____
_____
_____

After you watch a patient walk, and look at their leg length, you then should take a minute to observe their structure in stance. You need to step back 3 or 4 feet from the patient after you leg length examination, and look from front and back. You are looking for bow legs, knock knees, high arches, flat feet, and a variety of asymmetries.

Relaxed Calcaneal Stance Position
(key to understanding how the body is stacked up)

RCSP
(Right)_____
(Left)_____

One of the most crucial examination techniques is to bisect the center of the heel with the patient standing up and see if the heel is vertical, everted, or inverted. This is used in the initial evaluation for orthotic devices, and vital if you want to follow patients closely with the Inverted Orthotic Technique. It is used when orthotic devices are dispensed. The heel position is measured both with and without the orthotic devices to check if the orthotic correction was achieving the desired results. It is used in following the development of a growing child as you progress them over time through orthotic support, as you can be realistic with the parents of the progress or lack of progress. It is used in the pre-operative and post-operative evaluations of flat foot surgeries. It is used when you are just trying to understand the pronatory forces and if the patient is functioning fully pronated or subluxed even in stance.

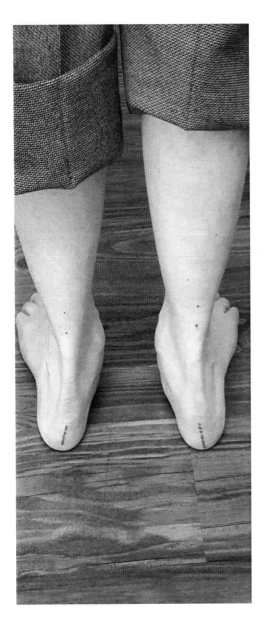

The posterior surface of the calcaneus or heel bone is usually flat and will be angled from posterior lateral to anterior medial on weight bearing. You must find the medial and lateral borders and put your fingers so they align superior to inferior. Your fingers should be flush with the middle of the calcaneus from superior to inferior, and clearly just on the medial and lateral edges off the posterior surface of the heel bone. Then make 3 points about one inch (2.5 cm) apart from superior to inferior bisecting the two sides as you are trying to represent the orientation of the heel bone. Draw a straight line downward connecting these three points. This can be done weight bearing or non-weight bearing with the patient in a prone position (one method will feel easier to you). When you are learning, do this and other measurements with others to see if you can agree. With non-weight bearing, please remember the posterior heel is best measured when completely perpendicular to your eyes, so angle the body to bring the posterior surface to this reference. The typical orientation of the posterior heel medial and lateral edges will be like a rectangle with straight parallel edges, or more rhomboid with divergent edges. Only a few percentages of heels are round which are very difficult to measure. After examining a few feet, students get the feel of this quite easily.

Once the heel is bisected extend the line as straight as possible another centimeter both superiorly and inferiorly. With the patient standing, look at the back of the heel and make sure your line looks straight all the way from top to bottom, and make sure the line looks like it matches what the heel looks like. By this I mean, when you stand several feet behind the patient, does the heel and line both look straight, both everted, or both inverted. With weight bearing, use an angle measuring device that is parallel with the posterior surface of the heel running posterior lateral to anterior medial. Now you are ready to measure the heel position to the ground. This measurement is typically done without orthotic devices, called the resting calcaneal stance position, or resting heel position. But, it is used to see how your orthotic devices, or surgery of some sort that should affect the heel, has done its job. An orthotic device, even with a deep heel cup, will not distort this line.

https://youtu.be/aPHi8gxF6Bc

What are common examples of the use and meaning of the relaxed calcaneal stance position, or simply the resting heel position? First of all, your definition of the heel as everted, inverted, or vertical speaks volumes. I think it is fine to just estimate how far from the heel neutral position it is (where the subtalar joint has been placed in neutral). This estimate will talk about compensations, and I like them to make sense. They can also mean injury, like when a heel is more inverted then it should be from peroneal tendon or lateral ankle ligament damage, or the heel is more everted than it should be from the advancement of posterior tibial tendon dysfunction stages or other subluxation problems. Some very common daily examples include:

- 7 degrees everted in resting with normal tibial and foot mechanics (should be a vertical heel)
- 7 degrees everted in resting with genu valgum noted and normal tibial and foot mechanics (pronation driven from extrinsic to foot)
- Vertical heel in resting with high tibial varum noted and normal foot mechanics (pronation needed to bring the front of the foot to the ground)
- 4 degrees inverted in resting with normal tibial and foot mechanics (should be vertical heel, something causing over supination)
- 3 degrees inverted in resting with tibial varum noted (need to find out if this a partially compensated rearfoot varus that can not get to a vertical heel position)
- 14 degrees everted heel in resting with 10 degrees forefoot varus and equinus forces (pronatory forces subluxing subtalar joint more than needed for forefoot varus correction only)

#68 Resting calcaneal stance position at least can help explain some of the symptoms patients complain of commonly. Match which of the 4 heel positions would produce pronatory symptoms or supinatory symptoms.
1. 10 degrees everted
2. Vertical
3. 8 degrees inverted
4. 3 degrees everted

(see page 139)

Neutral Calcaneal Stance Positions and Neutral Tibial Position

NCSP

(Right)_____

(Left)_____

Neutral Tibial Position

(Right)_____

(Left)_____

Neutral calcaneal stance position is measured like the resting or relaxed heel position, with the patient standing. It is helpful in categorizing patients with rearfoot varus deformities where the heel bisection is inverted while their subtalar joint is in neutral position. The measurement is taken from behind, and with the subtalar joint in neutral position. Neutral position is found when the head of the talus produces even pressure medially and laterally just in front of the ankle. You tell the patient is slowly move their medial arch up and down as you feel for this centered place in your fingers. This is where the foot is in direct alignment with the ankle. This is where the ankle is the most stable. It is where the foot and ankle are stacked properly. When is it useful? One of the most useful clinical applications is the degree difference of neutral to relaxed. This gives you reference on the amount of deformity you need to change to help someone when relaxed is everted. When the neutral position is moderate to highly inverted, it shows which patients need some inversion in their prescription.

Once you measure the neutral heel position, move up the leg to measure the neutral tibial position again bisecting the lower ⅓ of the leg. Most people have 4-5 degrees of tibial varum and therefore, can probably do well with the Inverted Orthotic Technique.

When this measurement was initially taught, it was a way to make the numbers work. You measured subtalar range of motion, and found subtalar joint neutral. You then added it to tibial position, and came up with a position that was ideal for patients to function at while walking. If you could design a pair of comfortable orthotic devices around this ideal position, you were going to help their symptoms greatly (in most cases, I still think this is fairly correct). You could check yourself to see if it matched your measured neutral heel resting position, and if not tried to make sense of the discrepancies. I believe now, at least in my practice, it is a great method to describe patients, and how they should work, and therefore find the reasons why they are not working well biomechanically. I want to know if they are vertical patients that evert for pronatory compensation, or inverted patients that supinate abnormally since they are already in an inverted position, or inverted patients (high tibial varum) that can not evert past perpendicular. These last patients at perpendicular or vertical are subluxed in a severely pronated position. I want to know if their biomechanics are influenced by their rearfoot or forefoot deformities, or some other factors like weak and tight muscles, running form, old injuries, etc. It makes me stop with each patient, get away from generalizations, and treat them individually which they deserve. So, I prefer utilizing neutral position and resting position measurements to help me get a sense of the patient's rearfoot frontal plane biomechanics. I feel that they are crucial measurements, not that it is important that they have specifically 7 or 8 or 10 degrees of tibial varum, but that they have high tibial varum that will cause their feet to do something to get the forefoot on the ground.

#69 You measure the patient's relaxed heel position and record 2 degrees inverted on the right and vertical on the left. We are taught that a vertical heel position is the most desirable and stable heel position, so you make orthotic devices to attempt to hold the foot at vertical on both sides. What foot deformity in general does not do well at a heel vertical position as an inverted heel position, and the Inverted Orthotic Technique to hold the foot at 5 degrees or so inverted would be better? Assume that the patient only has one biomechanical abnormality.
1. Forefoot Varus Deformity
2. Forefoot Valgus Deformity
3. Tibial Varum Deformity
4. Tibial Valgus Deformity
5. Metatarsus Primus Elevatus
6. Tight Achilles Tendons

(see page 139)

Functional Hallux Limitus

Functional Hallux Limitus (barefoot alone)
Right _____ Left_____
With Orthosis
Right_____ Left_____

As we walk, for normal propulsion, we need to be able to push off the ground powerfully by plantarflexing the first metatarsal and dorsiflexing the hallux at the time of heel lift. This is a crucial motion in gait. The gait becomes disturbed if we can not accomplish this feat, and various compensations occur like abductory twist or excessive out toeing or excessive lateral weight bearing. Typically, there is an insidious breakdown of the big toe joint. Functional Hallux Limitus implies the lack of big toe joint motion is functional not structural. Normal range of motion of dorsiflexion of the first metatarsal phalangeal joint is 75 degrees or greater. Less than 60 degrees of this motion is considered hallux limitus, and less than 30 degrees of this motion is considered hallux rigidus. This is measured by a goniometer or tractograph from the medial side of the foot bisecting first the medial side of the first metatarsal with one arm of the device and then the medial side of the hallux with the other arm of the device. The axis point is at the joint you are trying to measure. With functional hallux limitus, the hallux gets trapped against the ground and can not dorsiflex. The problem seems to be that the first metatarsal can not be free enough to plantarflex. The first metatarsal must plantarflex to allow the hallux to dorsiflex.

Stand the patient in their normal angle and base of gait resting position facing you. Grab under the big toe and try to dorsiflex the toe off the ground. If you can, you can also observe if the medial arch raises. If the joint is too jammed into the ground by overpronation, and medial shift of body weight, you will not be able to dorsiflex the hallux and raise the medial arch. I have some simple varus wedges in my office of ¼ inch or 4 degrees. When I find functional hallux limitus, I slide varus wedges under the heel, or put the patient on their orthotic devices, and check if the functional hallux limitus is eliminated.

This is a measurement that basically means that if a normal joint can be jammed up and restricted by simply standing with even weight on both feet, it probably will be worse in walking and running. This may or not be the case based on shoes, running style, walking mechanics, etc. In my practice, if a patient has big toe pain I want to know if that there is functional or structural problems, and since it basically is a sign of overpronation, I try to find out where the pronation is coming from and how to fix it if needed.

Functional hallux limitus can be a sign of significant problems that affect propulsion and the treatment of big toe joint pain. Functional hallux limitus was really popularized by Dr. Howard Dannenberg and his Sagittal Plane Blockade Theory. He said if we could not push through our feet we would get all sorts of problems including back pain. He designed the Kinetic Wedge and first ray cutouts along with the help of Langer Laboratory. Root was doing some of the same with narrow orthotic devices so as to not block first metatarsal plantarflexion. It is one of the biggest negative concerns with corrective orthotic devices attempting not to

block first metatarsal plantarflexion. When you dispense a pair of orthotic devices, the patient should feel that they can roll through their feet easily, and for pronators, that the weight is more in the center of the foot or at least partially onto the second metatarsal. In my design of the Inverted Technique, having the high point of correction under the first cuneiform navicular joint allows the first metatarsal to be free to plantar flex. The Kirby Skive was also designed to make sure the medial column was not overloaded.

When I dispense orthotic devices, or just in a pronation teaching moment to my students, I try to have my patients feel how their feet roll through the ball of the foot. I have them do one foot at a time, and they have to be walking normal. I want them to feel whether the weight is only on the first (too pronated), on the first and second (good), centered or 2nd and 3rd (probably best), or on 4 and 5 (too supinated). Because our feet are different, I need them to feel one at a time and see if they are the same or different. This way when they buy shoes in the future they will pick more stable ones by applying this same principle.

When performing the functional hallux limitus test, if the medial arch raises with any big toe joint motion (even if helped varus wedges or orthotic devices) it is called the Hubscher Maneuver. I will have a separate discussion below, but the functional hallux limitus test and Hubscher are done simultaneously.

#70 As you walk through your feet, you should have no restrictions in motion

forward. Typically orthotic devices make you more efficient by minimizing the side to side frontal plane motion, and directing motion more in the sagittal plane. Since we want a good push off at the big toe, should all our weight at push off be under the first metatarsal (yes or no)? _____
(see page 139)

Hubscher's Maneuver (and Jack's Test)

Hubscher Maneuver (and Jack's Test)
(Right)_____
(Left)_____

These maneuvers are both trying to see if your arch is flexible or rigid, and are actually part of the functional hallux limitus test in my office. With the Hubscher maneuver, you want to test if the patient can raise their flattened arch by moving the big toe upward. Is the arch collapse rigid or functional? It also shows if the big toe joint has some functional limitations as discussed above. If there some hallux limitus, you will have to eliminate the limitus before successfully performing this maneuver.

In life big toe joints get beat up. Most of my patients over fifty years old have some big toe joint degeneration (wear and tear). It was the advent of MRIs that really documented subtle joint wear and tear, sometimes years before you would see it on xray or they actually begin to hurt. It is no wonder that gout, which affects degenerative joints, picks on the big toe joint the most. The wear and tear is so common that most doctors pay little attention to it, even when the arthritic joint inflames occasionally.

Sometimes, the wear and tear is from old accidents, like sesamoid fractures unrelated to the patient's biomechanics. Yet, sometimes, the breakdown of the joint is highly predictable and easily remedied. One of the simplest maneuvers is Hubscher. The patient is standing barefoot, with equal weight on each foot, therefore 50% of normal weight. This is actually giving the patient the benefit of less pressure so they should be able to do the maneuver easily and most can. The big toe is then pushed upward from the bottom surface to see if the big toe can dorsiflexion and the medial arch can raise. When it can not, it is called functional hallux limitus (given that it can move fully in a relaxed non-weight bearing position). You can then test various modalities to see what can change the results and free up the big toe joint. Sometimes simple support like a 4 degree varus heel wedge is enough to free up the joint. Sometimes you need an orthotic device to have enough force to accomplish the task. Sometimes you need rearfoot support, medial arch support, and forefoot off weighting pads called dancer's pads or reverse Morton's extensions, to accomplish the task. So, the maneuver should be tied to what it takes to eliminate the functional hallux limitus you find. In my office, it is easy, at least in an initial evaluation to place varus wedges or dancer's padding, and see if the limitation of the big toe joint and medial arch height improves.

With Jack's test, you are also observing the medial arch to check the flexibility or rigidity. From a standing position, while observing the medial arch, have the patient do a heel raise and watch if the arch stays flat or improves. When I am designing an Inverted Orthotic Device, I need the arch to be flexible, to take on the new shape of the Device. If the arch is rigid, as I invert the foot, the midfoot will hang up around the 1st cuneiform leaving the big toe joint up in the air. While I have seen that naturally improve over time, it can make the orthotic device uncomfortable, and sweet spots are needed. I send many patients to physical therapy to attempt to loosen up the midfoot and heel valgus contractures (like in stage 3 and 4 PTTD). I also may have to support the foot distal to the 1st cuneiform with varus supports on top of the orthotic device or just make a Hybrid Inverted device extending the medial column support far under the first metatarsal, and sometimes to the base of the hallux. This then requires deep toe boxes like in the Ambulator extra depth shoe. Hopefully, slowly the foot can mold to my device, and the support distal to the 1st metatarsal base is gradually removed. The Jack's test before orthotic devices are made can help predict this path. The Jack's test with the orthotic device under the foot, looking from the front, can help you decide what modifications you need to perform to get the weight forward on to the first metatarsal head for stability.

#71 What test is crucial in a stage 4 PTTD where you are using the Inverted Orthotic Technique but the weight is hanging up on the first cuneiform area in determining modifications to make to help the first metatarsal bear weight?_____
(see page 139)

Single Leg Heel Raise Evaluation

Single Leg Heel Raise
(Right)_____
(Left)_____

This is one of the most significant evaluations because in its absence normal gait can not exist. The patient must be stable when doing the test, so one hand is resting on a solid surface, as we need this to be strength test not a balance test. Have the patient start with both feet on the ground, and lift one side off the ground. Then try to lift the heel of the support foot off the ground several times. Tell them to go slowly up and down. The gold standard of health is 25 repetitions. That feat can take a year to successfully perform by slowly adding more. I have my patients do it only in the evening before bed, and never through pain. Doing this exercise every other day is usually significant.

Why is this so important? A normal Achilles' tendon, the strongest tendon in the body, should be able to lift 4-5 times normal body weight rather easily. If the patient is having difficulty lifting their body weight doing a single heel raise, then normal activity will not happen. This recognition is most commonly made by those in sports medicine, but it is perhaps the most crucial made by podiatrists who deal with an aging population. The inability to do a single heel raise, if not reversed, while lead to a marked reduction of activity levels.

Single Leg Balancing

Single Leg Balance
(Right)_____
(Left)_____

Another very important indicator of leg health is the ability to balance on one foot barefoot for two minutes without holding on to a supporting surface. This is crucial in any fall program as our patient's age, but should be started earlier. It is again an evening task. Once you get good with your eyes open, and you have built up the strength to last 2 minutes with your knees slightly bent, you then have two choices to make it harder. You can try to balance with eyes open standing in the middle of a soft pillow, or you can try to close your eyes more and more for the 2 minutes. The next level on either is eyes open standing on a small rubber exercise balance disc (typically it has you elevated no more than an inch from the supporting surface). By making this exercise harder and harder, you are first building overall leg strength, and then developing the fast twitch muscles that will help prevent falls. Your reaction time will be sped up.

Single Leg Heel Lifts and Single Leg Balancing are a great start to stronger and more powerful legs. Overall ankle functional instability and weak achilles tendons are very detrimental to foot and leg health and vital part of our biomechanical evaluation.

Patient Lying Prone:

We are finished our gait and weight bearing evaluations, so now we need to lay the patient down starting on their stomachs (prone).

Ankle Joint Dorsiflexion Non-Weight Bearing (why not Weight Bearing?) (key to finding both equinus forces and hypermobility problems, both leading to ankle weakness)

AJDF
(Right) straight_____bent_____
(Left) straight_____bent_____

Ankle joint dorsiflexion with the knee extended and flexed will tell us a lot about the tightness or weakness (over flexibility) of the gastrocnemius and soleus muscles. These are the two muscles that make up the achilles tendon, the strongest and most powerful and possibly the most influential tendon in the body. Tightness and weakness can have severe effects on the knee, ankle, arch, and metatarsals. They directly affect the ankle and knee joint (gastrocnemius crosses the knee), but indirectly affect every structure in the foot. Being able to measure the overall tightness, and seeing how it correlates to the normal Achilles force-length curve, is a very powerful help for so many injuries including all Achilles problems, shin splints, ankle problems, all calf problems, all foot problems, etc. It is probably influential in most lower extremity injuries to at least some degree.

Achilles' tendon flexibility measurement (called ankle joint dorsiflexion) is done along the lateral side of the foot and leg. One arm of a measuring device (called goniometer or tractograph) is aligned straight through the lateral malleolus and the fifth metatarsal head, and one arm is aligned through the lateral malleolus to the head of the fibula. The axis of the goniometer is at the ankle joint laterally. You then grab the foot and slightly supinate the subtalar joint and longitudinal axis of the midtarsal joint by inverting the first metatarsal. You must maintain that subtalar joint position while you ask the patient to help you pull the foot into a more flexed ankle position. Ideally, as the patient pulls their foot up with a stable leg, the angle created for the gastrocnemius tightness (knee extended) is 10-12 degrees, and for the soleus tightness (knee flexed) is 15-18 degrees. In my travels, I have found some doctors who supinate more than this so will get a normal flexibility of 0-5 degrees. I have also found those you allow the subtalar joint to pronate while measuring and will get more degrees as normal. I believe if you practice this technique on 10 individuals, the average should be 10 degrees with the knee extended and 15 degrees with the knee flexed, with some being tighter and some being looser. If your average is less or more than this by many degrees, you should go back and read through the steps listed above. In teaching this vital technique, I have occasionally found that some doctors will reliably get 5 degrees or so more or less dorsiflexion than I that is consistent. I tell them to just accept their average as normal, and treat the patient based on that. One such doctor said all of his patients had tight achilles. So, his 0 degrees was 10 degrees to me, and he had to adjust accordingly.

What does this mean? When we take a step, for smooth transfer of weight forward, our ankles must dorsiflex. At the middle of midstance, our body's weight is directly over our foot, and our ankle joint is at neutral position or 0 degrees dorsiflexed. Just as we lift our heels off the ground at the end of midstance, the ankle has now dorsiflexed 10 degrees with the knee straight fairly straight. As the heel lifts off the ground, we begin the propulsive phase of gait, with ankle plantar flexion and knee flexion preparing to lift the foot and toes off the ground. So, for a smooth gait, the ankle should bend 10 degrees at a time when the knee is fairly straight. This is the definition of normal ankle joint dorsiflexion. If we have less than 10 degrees, we have an equinus deformity, and if we have more than 12 degrees, we are over flexible. The measurements are accurate within 2 degrees, and change 2-3 degrees more flexible from morning to night. The measurement is very reliable with the same examiner, so you should be able to follow patients and the changes with flexibility programs. If you measure the next 10 patients the same way and your average is 8-12, you are doing it right. If your average is greater than 15 or less than 5, then you are measuring them differently than I. If you measure consistently, which is the most important point, you still will be able to follow the trend of the achilles towards more flexibility or more tightness. It will work. Most of my patients have normal flexibility, so if most or all of your patients are tight or loose, I would review the examination with a colleague or fellow student.

This is a perfect time to discuss the force-length curve of tendons where the normal lower extremity tendons (Achilles, quadriceps, and hamstrings) have been extensively measured. Force is the vertical axis and length of the tendon is the horizontal axis. The normal length of a tendon, where it is considered not tight or not too flexible, is called the Resting Length, or Normal Physiological Length. If the gastrocnemius is normal at ankle joint dorsiflexion of 10-12 degrees, it means it is too tight at less than 10 degrees, and it means it is too loose at greater than 12 degrees. The same is true for the soleus at 15-18 degrees normal, under 15 degrees means it is too tight to some degree, and over 18 degrees means it is too loose to some degree. The Force Length curve argues that away from its Normal Physiological Length that any tendon becomes weaker. When a tendon is tighter than it should be, aka muscle-bound, the actin and myosin filaments are too bound up, producing less of a neurological charge, and therefore less of a powerful contraction. The tighter a tendon is away from its normal, the weaker it becomes. I have found this so true and it has helped me manage many injuries with this knowledge. The same is true when the tendon is looser than normal, it becomes weaker, or more stretched out. Here the actin and myosin filaments are not in as close contact with each other, thus less of a neurological charge, thus weaker in function.

There are so many examples of how this is important, but I will just mention one here. A patient presented to the office with 2 years of chronic Achilles tendinitis. Previous MRIs and ultrasound had not found any problem. The treatment had been for Achilles stretching three times a day, orthotic devices for heel stability, icing, some physical therapy for flexibility, strength, and anti-inflammatory, and when there was no improvement, some acupuncture and a surgical opinion to lengthen the tight tendon. The Achilles' tendon at presentation definitely had slight swelling, but not like the swelling of tendinosis. The patient could not do 25 single heel raises (my gold standard of Achilles strength). When I measured his ankle joint dorsiflexion, I found 29 degrees with the knee extended, and 34 degrees with the knee flexed. Who knows what the flexibility was when he started, but his stretching 3 or more times a day for 2 years had probably gone the wrong direction. When I told him I want heel lifts and shoes with heel elevation nonstop for the next month with no stretching, I could tell he really did not believe me. I also wanted pain free 2 positional Achilles strengthening every day, since it would take a while to do single leg heel raises pain free, but two positional was fine to start with. After the first month, he was beginning to feel symptomatically better, and his measurements had reduced to 22 and 29. By the end of the next month, he had almost no pain, and his measurements 17 and 26. He passed the 30 minutes of pain-free fast walking test at 2 and ½ months, so I started him on a walk-run program, and started single leg 2 positional heel raises each evening. By the end of the fourth month, he was running 30 minutes pain-free, and his measurements were 14 and 24. I told him he was still too flexible, but out of the woods. I discouraged any form of stretching for another couple months and made sure he warmed up well walking or on a stationary bike before running. I think in general, since he commented that his flexibility had been measured in the past and found to be normal, that once health care providers get to 10 degrees with the knee extended they may stop measuring and not complete the exact measurement therefore missing over flexibility.

I also want to discuss ankle joint dorsiflexion measurement weight bearing. It is possible to do this measurement in very stable orthotics that do not allow for any pronation compensation. Weight bearing has much more force to pronate the foot allowing the talus to plantarflex within the ankle, subtalar joint and midtarsal joint and therefore allowing more forward excursion of the tibia. A large study has to be done comparing the weight bearing to non weight bearing examinations, but I can not see how the orthotic part will be worked out. It is so very hard to do any orthotic based research project. And, if you just allow the foot to pronate while measuring, the varying degrees of increased pronation will make any study useless. You must create standards for reproducibility, and non weight bearing has passed the reproducibility tests historically. I know if I have someone that is too tight, and I measure their flexibility, that I will be accurate within a few degrees, therefore in a month or 6 months, I can reproduce the same measurement and check progress. This is because I measure the motion the same way every time and the test is very reproducible for the same examiner at least.

#72 A patient presents with achilles tendinitis and metatarsalgia. The achilles tightness is measured with the knee straight and flexed. Ankle joint dorsiflexion was -2 degrees and 19 degrees. What muscle is tight?_____
(see page 139)

Forefoot Deformities
(forefoot varus feet function different than forefoot valgus feet, and will that influence treatment?)

Forefoot Deformity
(Right)_____ (Left)_____
After mobilization (if varus)
(Right)_____ (Left) _____

Forefoot deformities are the relationships of the front of the foot to the back of the foot in a non weight bearing position. They are the alignment variations that define the front of the foot as the neutral and relaxed subtalar joint positions can define the back of the foot. They are measured with the patient in a prone position by placing the subtalar joint in neutral position and maximally pronating the midtarsal joints. This will be the same way to take the impression cast for custom orthotics with the subtalar neutral and the midtarsal joints maximally pronated. Some prefer to cast supine and some prefer prone, but they tend to get the same results unless there is a very loose unstable midtarsal joint. Appendix 9 will go over impression casting in subtalar joint neutral with its variations. I know that the impression taken with suspension casting is very different with foam box or puddle casting, so making treatment decisions when these casts are used can not be easily done. The common everted forefoot deformities are forefoot valgus, plantar flexed first ray, forefoot evertus, and the common inverted forefoot deformities are forefoot varus, plantar flexed fourth and/or fifth rays, and forefoot supinatus. Some are structural deformities that will not change, some are combination deformities that will change some, and some are functional deformities that can completely disappear with the right treatment. If forefoot deformities influence the making of your orthotic devices, I recommend carefully noting the deformity measured on the table and in the cast (should be within 2 degrees although more discussion in Appendix 9), and re-measuring every 2 years. If the measurement changes more than the 2 acceptable degrees, new casts are needed.

When you measure forefoot varus, it is only the surgeons in my mind that need to know if the alignment is really due to a plantarflexed 4 or 5 metatarsal. I will treat it the same as forefoot varus or supinatus, meaning it is the same alignment I have to

deal with in an orthotic device of an inverted forefoot on the rearfoot. It is very important to know if it is a forefoot supinatus, since some or all of the troubling inverted angulation can be removed by mobilization of the forefoot on the rearfoot. You hold the heel steady, typically after 5 minutes of a heat pack on top of the foot, and you attempt to reduce the supinatus with forefoot eversion several times. Dr. Paul Scherer popularized the notion of putting pressure on the first metatarsal head from the top while casting supine to plantarflex and evert to remove any supinatus. I mention it for completeness, but have not used it. I use the mobilization technique. It is important to note that if you measure a forefoot varus angulation, you can attempt mobilization before casting. Forefoot supinatus occurs with heel eversion jamming the forefoot into a functional varus position by primarily supinating the longitudinal axis of the midtarsal joint. If you find a forefoot varus, without a resting heel everted position, there can be no supinatus deformity.

Forefoot varus (where the first metatarsal is aligned higher than the 2nd, and down the line, with the 5th metatarsal the lowest when you strike the ground), will force the heel to evert (pronate) to bring the metatarsals in line with the ground. Technically 5 degrees of forefoot varus alone should place your heel 5 degrees everted, but with a lot of other forces, it is at least a pronatory problem.

Measuring the forefoot deformity before and after mobilization is done with forefoot varus feet. Forefoot varus feet, or accurately termed inverted forefoot deformities, can be structural or functional or combination. If you have a forefoot varus, measured with the patient prone in subtalar joint neutral position, the forefoot will be inverted to the rearfoot (measured to a line perpendicular to the heel bisection). However, there is a functional mimic called forefoot supinatus, that can be resolved with mobilization or after prolonged correction of pronation. The forefoot supinatus is created by the ground reactive force when your heel everts. With heel eversion past perpendicular, the forefoot is chronically jammed upward in the frontal plane causing the forefoot varus imitator. Manipulation of the forefoot varus prior to casting is done with an eversion force of the forefoot and with the heel held stable. The forefoot varus deformity is measured before and after mobilization to see if some supinatus was reduced. Commonly, a 12 degree inverted forefoot deformity, if full or part functional, can be reduced to 6 degrees or less. So, 50% correction is common in this functional problem. Some doctors use a 10 minute heating pack prior to mobilization to help loosen the foot.

Why is this important? As you will see when we talk about orthotic corrections (appendix 8), forefoot varus angulations are not an easy task to support correctly. The higher the forefoot varus in the impression cast, the more modification is needed in the positive cast correction. This is not true in forefoot valgus feet. In forefoot varus over 4-5 degrees, if you were to use the Root Balancing system, you would potentially block first ray plantarflexion at push off. Definitely over 5 degrees you will have to reduce the support to the first and 2nd metatarsal shafts with a modified Root correction, or change techniques entirely by changing to the Inverted Orthotic Technique. Appendix 8 describes all these orthotic modifications. So, if you can mobilize the foot to reduce some of that forefoot inverted positioning when there is silent forefoot supinatus present, you make the orthotic device more stable, and you will have less modifications to do.

Therefore, you have already measured resting heel position as one of your initial measurements. Only if it is everted is there an opportunity for supinatus. If you measure an everted heel, and you measure an inverted forefoot deformity, that deformity may be forefoot varus or forefoot supinatus. You can then mobilize the forefoot on the rearfoot, even if you are not going to take an impression cast at that time, to see if some of the inverted position reduces. If it does, prior to casting for sure, use a ten minute hot pack prior to the mobilization.

In honor of recently passed Dr. Paul Scherer from ProLab USA, if there is a forefoot supinatus suspected, he taught practitioners to plantar flex the first metatarsal when casting. I have never done this, but the principle is sound. As explained in the Appendix 9 on Impression Casting, one of the problems with supine casting is that if there is laxity in the midfoot, any forefoot inverted positioning can be removed by the invisible pull of gravity. Prone casting is preferable in cases of ligamentous laxity when the exact forefoot to rearfoot relationship is needed in forefoot varus cases.

#73 The Inverted Orthotic Technique can be used in every pronatory case, including the excessive pronation caused by forefoot varus/forefoot supinatus situations which compensate by heel eversion. Most laboratories do a wonderful job supporting forefoot varus feet of minor degrees (less than 5), but higher degrees of inverted forefoot deformities when corrected cause too much first ray blockage limiting propulsion. If you measure 10 degrees of forefoot varus, but manipulation reduces the measurement to 5 degrees, what would be pouring angle of an Inverted Orthotic Device? _____
(see page 139)

First Ray Range of Motion
(do you have a plantar flexed first metatarsal, a metatarsus primus elevatus, does the sesamoids have range of motion to get out of the way?)

First Ray Range of Motion
Right (Up)_____ (Down)_____
Left (Up)_____ (Down)_____

First ray range of motion, and really the evaluation of the metatarsal arch, is very crucial in any forefoot surgery, and conservative treatment in this area (for example sesamoid fractures). We measure first ray range of motion, with the same reference point as the forefoot deformities, with the subtalar joint in a neutral position and the midtarsal joint maximally pronated.

When motion is measured, you are relating the motion of one part to a stable reference point. This is like ankle joint dorsiflexion where the foot moves on a stable leg. Here, with first ray range of motion, the second metatarsal is stable and the first metatarsal is moved in relationship to it. Ideally, the first metatarsal moves equally above (5 mm) and below (5 mm) the second metatarsal head. In a plantar flexed first metatarsal, there is more plantar motion or it is in a more plantar position overall. In a metatarsus primus elevatus, there is more dorsal motion or it is in a more dorsal position overall. The average excursion, whether it is more up or down, defines the deformity. Since all of our weight walking ends up through the hallux, these are vitally important measurements. We need a first metatarsal to go below the plane of the second metatarsal for a good push off. In push off, the second metatarsal is the stabilizer with the first metatarsal pushing off the ground. If the first metatarsal is elevated to the second, and can not push off, three things tend to happen:

1. The weight remains lateral with too much pressure on the lesser metatarsals
2. The weight abnormally shifts to an unstable first metatarsal causing late midstance or propulsive phase pronation
3. The gait is apropulsive without push off

#74 The first metatarsal head is the end of the medial column. It is the third leg of our tripod of support. An elevated first metatarsal is disaster to that medial column stability, and if present, we need to support under the first metatarsal head to bring the ground up to it. What is this support called?

_____

(see page 139)

Subtalar Joint Neutral Position
(are they hypermobile, limited with perhaps a tarsal coalition, do they have range of motion to obtain a vertical heel in stance, and do they function around subtalar neutral?)

STJ NP
(Right) Inv___ Ev___ NP___
(Left) Inv____ Ev____ NP___
Total ROM - ⅔ ROM =Neutral from Max Eversion

First of all, this is the second ideal position of the foot concerning how centered the heel is to the lower leg. We have already discussed how the heel is aligned to the ground in neutral calcaneal stance position. It is all about reference points. The ideal stability of the lower extremity has the heel bone vertical (not inverted or everted), and the alignment of the heel to leg neither inverted or everted. But, we do not live in a perfect world. There are numerous varus and valgus deformities of the tibia, or just various tibial relationships to the ground due to knee alignment issues, and numerous varus and valgus deformities of the calcaneus, and then numerous varus and valgus subtalar joint neutralities. We are either centering the heel near verticality to the ground, inverted to the ground, or everted to the ground to make the patient

more stable. It is knowing when everted or inverted to the ground makes sense for maximum stability that we go through these tests. This measurement helps us understand what we are doing to achieve stability. I also see so many subluxed subtalar joints or coalitions, that this measurement will not work for.

Subtalar joint neutral position defines the relationship of the heel to the stationary talus and is very useful in differentiating the variations and how those change treatment. It is utilized in my practice to get a feel of the motion: normal with about 30 degrees, hypermobile with more than 30 degrees, and limited as in cases of tarsal coalition. The subtalar joint neutral position is simply the position of the heel bone in the subtalar joint where it lines up with the talus. When you move the subtalar joint around the stationary talus, neutral position felt or can be calculated as total range of motion minus 2/3s of that overall motion. These are the degrees from maximal eversion (since the rule is ⅔ of subtalar joint motion is supinatory) that is called subtalar joint neutral. For example, in a perfect world, the subtalar joint has 20 degrees of inversion and 10 degrees of eversion for a total of 30 degrees. If neutral is 30 degrees minus 20 from maximal eversion(1/3 total), then neutral is neither inverted or everted from the talus. In another example, if the range of motion is 15 inversion and 15 eversion, 30 minus 20 means that the neutral subtalar position is 5 everted. This is how we define calcaneal varus or valgus by its relationship to the talus. I actually look at the degrees some, but prefer to measure the position by feel which is mentioned below.

Sports, like ballet, that have studied this position for centuries know its importance. When you are en pointe in ballet, a pronated position from neutral is called winging, and a supinated position from neutral is called sickling. These mechanical flaws in a ballet dancer, functioning away from the ideal neutral centered position of the ankle joint, are disastrous in terms of injuries. When the subtalar joint's alignment is neutral, there are even forces that go up from the foot to the ankle to the knee. It is an extremely stable position needing very little muscle power to maintain its position for prolonged standing. A general rule of podiatry has been that it is an ideal position of stability when this neutral subtalar joint position corresponds to a vertical heel position. Since this only occurs sometimes, due to the variances in subtalar joints, and due to the common presence of various rearfoot varus deformities, the common trend in making someone stable by getting their heel position close to vertical may not be correct. I think heel verticality, not subtalar joint neutral is the most common treatment goal now practiced in podiatry. In my work in biomechanics and sports medicine, the 2 positions I try to obtain commonly in treating patients is either heel verticality or an inverted heel due to tibial varum or some shin, knee, and hip problem needing even more inversion force away from heel verticality. The Inverted Orthotic Device commonly uses an inversion force with the orthotic device to take an everted position of the heel, and bring it towards verticality. I have used up to 12 degrees of inversion in a functional foot orthotic device just to get the heel to a vertical heel position (from an everted position). However, you can use that same inversion force to take a foot from slightly everted to 6-8 degrees inverted if it helps their alignment.

So now do we find it? I was taught two methods by Dr. Merton Root himself. With the patient in prone, we first bisect the heel as previously described and move the heel medially and laterally around the stationary talus and tibia. This should be pure subtalar joint motion. Then with our other hand, we bring our fingers over to the medial and lateral sides of the talus in front of the malleoli. We move the heel medially and laterally slowly while we feel for a place where the talus is even on both sides of the joint. When the subtalar joint is pronated, you can feel more of the talus medial. When the subtalar joint is supinated, you can feel more of the talus lateral. Once you get that even feeling of the talus on both sides, you now can measure the neutral position directly and see if it corresponds to your ⅓ and ⅔ formula.

The other method is a gentle motion of the subtalar joint with an ounce of force on the forefoot. Again the patient is prone and the heel bisected. You can feel a gentle arch created by the joint axis. Start with the subtalar joint in full inversion and then let the heel evert slowly. As you move through the arch of motion, you can perceive where the drop down from inversion becomes the gentle pull up into eversion. That is subtalar joint neutral.

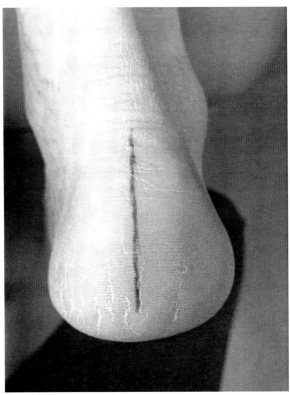

When do I use subtalar joint neutral position in my day to day podiatry practice:

1. You place the subtalar joint in neutral with your impression casts.
2. You place the subtalar joint in neutral position to measure forefoot deformities and metatarsal alignment.
3. If subtalar joint neutral positioning is the ideal, knowing whether it is vertical, everted, or inverted to the tibia or ground can help you understand how shoes work, orthotic devices work, or wedges work.

A common example is a patient who has bowlegs. Everyone can see that bowlegs means a high degree of tibial varum, thus rearfoot varus. This particular patient had long standing tarsal tunnel syndrome with some degenerative back issues. Their nerve conduction study showed a problem with the posterior tibial nerve running through the tarsal tunnel, but also enough low back disease, that at some point both back and tarsal tunnel surgeries were being contemplated. The patient had some handsome looking orthotic devices that seemed to help some set the heel at a vertical position. After evaluating the patient for a biomechanical opinion, and doing the relaxed calcaneal stance position and the subtalar joint neutral position, it was obvious where one of the problems lie. The relaxed position was 4 inverted, and the neutral subtalar position was 1 degrees inverted. With 7 degrees of tibial varum, the neutral calcaneal stance position was 8 inverted. The patient had 15 degrees total range of motion 11 inversion and 4 degrees eversion. His neutral subtalar joint position calculation was (15-10 =5 degree change from maximal eversion). When I just measured the neutral position from feeling the joint more, I measured one degree different only. An orthotic device made to hold the heel at vertical (resting heel position in the orthotic device was 1 degree inverted), a position that the patient could not obtain, was placing a terrible pronatory force on the subtalar joint and tarsal tunnel. I had many options: standard Root orthotic device set at 7 degree inverted (2 above most pronated), standard Root orthotic device set at 3 degrees inverted with 3 mm Kirby skive, or a 25 degree Inverted Orthotic device which puts the same 5 degree inversion force. I used the Inverted Technique of 25 degrees, and later set the inversion to 35 degrees with Kirby skive after only partial improvement. This mechanical treatment gave some wonderful help, and was coupled with some topical nerve gel, neural flossing, TENS unit, and a slight ⅛ inch varus wedge to the outsole of his shoes. One of the sad things with his initial history, although it helped in my treatment pain, was that early in his treatment he had noted a significant improvement with a pair of shoes broken down to the lateral side, and had told doctors of this. One health care provider had given him some sort of varus wedge also which had helped. But, by the time he got custom orthotics, the vertical heel position was forced on him with each step. I followed this patient for awhile, all his tarsal tunnel symptoms resolved except for a flare after a beach vacation where he wore flip flops for several weeks. He did eventually have some sort of back surgery, but not for his tarsal tunnel.

#75 Subtalar range of motion was 21 inversion and 12 eversion. There are 4 degrees of tibial varum. There is a 10 degree forefoot valgus causing contact phase supination. The resting heel position is 5 inverted. What is his NCSP? _____
(see page 139)

Patient Lying Supine:

Subtalar Joint Axis

Subtalar Joint Axis
Right_____
Left_____

Dr. Kevin Kirby, podiatrist out of Sacramento, California, popularized the concept in the early 1990's of variations in the subtalar axis and a technique to identify that position. He discussed that if your orthotic device, or wedge, did not have enough power on the medial side of the subtalar joint axis you would never stop the dangerous force of pronation. His Kirby Skive, and my Inverted Technique, have tried to place a force to decelerate subtalar joint pronation when excessive. The same is true with a laterally deviated subtalar joint axis that must be stabilized with a lateral Kirby Skive, Feehery cuboid support, Denton modification, maximal everted forefoot deformity support, and Fettig modification to the Inverted Orthotic Technique to stop supination tendencies. I refer you to Dr. Kirby's article on Subtalar Joint Axis evaluation.

I think it is important to feel the subtalar joint move. Move it gently through its range of motion. Is that motion smooth? Is that motion limited, normal, or excessive? Is the motion normal triplanar, or more transverse? High pitched subtalar joint axis give more transverse plane motion, and that can be hard to control with a standard Root orthotic device. Most of my high axis subtalar joint patients get the Inverted Technique due to the transverse plane pronatory motion.

Midtarsal Joint Range of Motion

MTJ ROM
(Right)_____
(Left)_____

With the patient supine, place the subtalar joint in neutral, hold the heel firmly to keep you from deviating from subtalar joint neutral, and move the midtarsal joint. Do this to the next one hundred patients and see the variations. Some of the patients barely move at all, some have more transverse plane abduction and adduction, and some have excessive motion where the joint seems not to have any firm end points (I tell these patients that designing an orthotic for them may be like nailing jello to a wall). This is the quality of motion of the midtarsal joint and can have tremendous variability. The more stable the midtarsal joint, the easier for you to stabilize with an orthotic device. The less stable the midtarsal joint, the harder it will be (an art project). The more transverse plane it moves, the more lateral phalanges on the orthotic to block closed kinetic chain forefoot abduction on the rearfoot and the only reason you may use the Inverted Orthotic Technique. Again, this is a simple observation, but if you can spot the challenging patients, it will help in your approach to them.

#76 If a joint axis produces more transverse plane motion, the axis is oriented more vertical, thus considered a vertical axis if that is the dominant motion. An axis in the transverse plane mainly, would produce motion mainly in the _____plane. (see page 139)

Ankle Inversion, Eversion, and Dorsiflexion Strength
Further Strength Testing
(Right) Inversion_____

(Left) Inversion_____
(Right) Eversion_____
(Left) Eversion_____
(Right) Dorsiflexion_____
(Left) Dorsiflexion_____

Biomechanics is as much about strength as it is about deformities and instabilities. A great strength program is key to helping patients become more stable. There are 4 directions of motion to develop strength and test for weaknesses in the ankle. We have already covered the achilles or plantar flexion strength. The other 3 directions to be tested and strengthened when need be are inversion, eversion, and dorsiflexion. These can be further broken down to 7 directions to isolate with each direction further isolating an individual muscle. These 7 directions are:

1. Inversion in ankle neutral--anterior tibial tendon
2. Inversion in ankle plantarflexion--posterior tibial tendon
3. Eversion in ankle dorsiflexion--peroneus tertius
4. Eversion in ankle neutral--peroneus longus
5. Eversion in ankle plantarflexion--peroneus brevis
6. Dorsiflexion in subtalar neutral--extensor hallucis longus
7. Dorsiflexion in subtalar pronation--extensor digitorum longus

Of course each direction will give us some overlap, but it is important to be able to isolate muscles for strength testing and rehabilitation.

In general, I do the testing and the physical therapist does the rehabilitation, but it is important to follow the progress of your patients. I want to see if the physical therapist has the patient on global functional and isolation exercises. The only types of strengthening exercises that I use are:

1. Active range of motion (with gravity)
2. Active range of motion (against gravity)
3. Isometric (same length)
4. Progressive Resistance
5. Isotonic (same weight)
6. Functional (where hold groups get strengthened together)
7. Isokinetic (same speed, but rarely used)

The general rules of strengthening that I have learned:

1. Start strengthening an injured area as soon as possible
2. There should be no pain with the exercises, or at least, no pain after the exercises are completed
3. All strengthening programs should include isolation exercises for the individual muscle injured or the closest muscles to the injured area
4. Each month follow visit should record an improvement of strength
5. It is important to find out where the patient's strength is so that the appropriate level of strengthening is being used (progressive resistive vs isotonic vs isometric, etc.)

#77 Which one of these exercises would not help someone with severe pronation?
1. Posterior tibial tendon
2. Soleus muscle
3. Internal hip rotators
4. Peroneus longus
5. Piriformis

(see page 139)

Appendix 6: Pronation Control (Simple to Complex)

Over the Counter Inserts for Pronation Control

There has been an explosion of inserts on the market that almost or do claim that they can decide as well as an expert what is the best biomechanics for the consumer. Yes, over the counter inserts can help by supplying some support and/or cushion, but they can also be very detrimental to the care of the patient. When hit with an injury, patients read online what helps and start checking off the list of helpful items. They get improper inserts, do improper stretches, use heat not ice or vice versa, change to improper shoes, get improper health care advice or treatments, and the injuries get worse. How often does it happen? They fill my office daily. Even when I do everything right, there are so many components to helping someone, and so many ways to go wrong also, it is a humbling journey to help people at times. So, ads or YouTube videos that claim 99% relief of heel pain if you buy this product, or do this exercise, I am not a fan of. Yes, patients still need their podiatrist.

Yet, I love to direct my patients to get several of the over the counter inserts that I can customize (be control over) to help a problem. I standardly use Sole and Powerstep products, which have no plastic, so I can customize to their needs and sensitivities. I typically increase the medial arch, but sometimes have to lower it. I typically varus wedge the insert, but sometimes have to valgus wedge it. I

sometimes soften the heel or raise the heel, or cut out the toe area or entire ball of the foot. My adjustments to these inserts follow my logic with custom made inserts: try to make the patient more stable and more comfortable.

Varus Wedges for Pronation Control

Varus wedges, also called runner's wedges, have been a crucial device in sports medicine and orthopedic practices. For the average size patient, 1/16th inch of wedge is equivalent to 1 degree of varus change of the foot into more of an inverted position. Therefore, it is quite common that varus wedges of ¼ inch or ⅜ inch are used to produce 4 or 6 degrees of inversion force at the heel to control excessive pronation forces, or invert the heel for better rear foot varus support, or to relax the structures in the medial ankle like the tarsal tunnel, or when treating the knee you can attempt to open up the lateral knee compartment when there is an injury, or just try to stabilize internal rotation forces medially. Varus wedges of course control the heel position at heel strike and have less power to help a forefoot runner, or any force in the propulsive phase of gait, therefore varus wedges for runners or propulsive phase pronation must include the forefoot. Varus wedges have been utilized in my practice for years in helping standing pronation complaints. They are simple to make, and variations can be made longer to have more of an effect. Varus wedges act on many mechanical layers: position shift, slowing of pronation motion, off weighting an area like the lateral knee joint, increasing the medial heel, ankle, and knee weight load, and in general stabilizing the lower leg.

Taping in Pronation Control

The J strap for pronation control, or inversion support, with coverall and leukotape is the king of taping procedures. It is utilized for very important problems like tarsal tunnel related to pronation, posterior tibial tendon dysfunction, and healing after flatfoot procedures while the orthotics and strength gain is changing. This taping works on the heel position and subtalar or ankle joint pronation.
https://youtu.be/AcSSyBfFocE
The classic Low Dye with its many versions helps mainly with the midtarsal joint part of foot pronation, and some subtalar joint. It is finding out when these different corrections are needed that is crucial. In my practice, the classic low dye has been replaced by Quick Tape from supportthefoot.com, but I am sure that there are advantages to each. If I do not get the relief I desire with taping, I experiment with all the variations out there.
https://youtu.be/shK6SyUuPl4

Strengthening and Flexibility in Pronation Control

Excessive foot pronation is an internal rotation torque that can pick on various structures at anytime when the motion is too much, too fast, too long in duration, or ends up leaving the body in poor alignment.

Stability shoes, simple activity changes, taping for pronation support, and corrective inserts, can all help minimize the stress and prevent re-occurrences. Strengthening exercises used to combat the stress of pronation on the body are: metatarsal doming, posterior tibial, anterior tibial, and peroneus longus, gastrocnemius and soleus, lateral hamstring and external hip rotators. Stretching exercises that seem to help with ease pronatory forces are: Achilles and plantar fascia, medial hamstring, and internal hip rotators.

Custom Orthotic Devices in Pronation Control

With 27 injuries and pain patterns associated with the complexity of some type of abnormal foot pronation (see appendix 1), either the amount of motion, the speed of the motion, the timing of the motion, the overall position that the pronation leaves you at, and the primary direction of motion in the frontal, sagittal, or transverse planes, it is then important to understand the powerful components of a custom made functional foot orthotic device. I use custom orthotic devices when my evaluation reveals a complexity that other forms of pronation control will not address adequately, when I am dealing with a growing child I want to insure good growth and a perfect match to their feet, and in chronic pain syndromes where I do not want to take the chance that an over the counter device will help subjectively and I could do it better for them. In appendix 8, I breakdown the types of orthotics and all the prescription variables commonly used in Podiatry. I will save the discussion until then.

Checklist of Available Modalities to Help with Pronation
1. OTC Shoe Inserts that can be customized
2. Varus Wedges
3. Varus Midsole Wedging
4. Varus Outsole Wedging
5. J Strap Taping
6. Low Dye or Quick Tape
7. Strengthening Exercises
8. Stretching Exercises
9. Shoe Changes to More Stable
10. High Topped Boot
11. Custom Orthotic Devices

#78 When you are helping someone with one or many symptoms of excessive pronation, which of the following should be considered commonly helpful?
1. Varus heel wedges
2. Over The Counter Arch supports
3. Quick Tape from supportthefoot.com
4. Leukotape for heel eversion control
5. Low Dye Taping
6. Motion Control Shoes
7. Custom Foot Orthotic Devices
8. All of the Above

(see page 139)

Appendix 7: Role of Weak and Tight Muscles

Stretching Principles

In treating the lower extremity, it is very important to emphasize stretching of the most important muscles groups: plantar arch, calf, quadriceps, hamstrings, iliotibial band, hip flexors, hip extensors, and hip adductors. Of these 8 groups, there are variations that are important, like separating the stretch for the gastrocnemius and soleus while doing calf stretches. Here are the basic principles I teach. If patients learn a few at first, you can build onto these principles so that they become smart stretchers. The 14 general stretching tips are:

1. Hold each stretch for 30 to 60 seconds and repeat twice. My trainer uses the principle for anyone over 30, hold one second for each year you have been alive.
2. Alternate between sides while stretching.
3. Do not bounce while stretching, prolonged hold.
4. Deep breath while stretching to get oxygen to the tissue (one deep breath per 6 seconds).
5. Stretching before activities should be done after a light warm up (do not stretch cold).
6. Stretching after a workout will gain you the most since the tissue is heated up.
7. If one side of the body is tighter, do twice as many on that side to gradually seek balance.
8. If you want to gain flexibility, stretch 3 times a day whether you work out that day or not.
9. If you want to just maintain flexibility, stretch once daily.
10. Never stretch through pain.
11. Make sure when stretching your body is stable.
12. Stretch the tissue in varying positions to see if you find some tightness.
13. If you are sore, and you can find a stretch that helps, you are on your way towards getting better.
14. If stretching the sore area makes no difference, you may be stretching a tendon that is too flexible (have it measured), or the pain that you think is from tightness is more inflammatory or neurological, or the problem is much deeper than the more superficial tendon.

When someone is an overpronator, and you are utilizing the Inverted Technique to fight that pronation, it is crucial that there is no achilles and hamstring tightness. These equinus producers can cause excessive arch pressure which will fight the inversion force placed into the orthotic device. Recognition and elimination of equinus can make for an easier time controlling pronation forces.

#79 Which of the following is not a method of gaining calf/achilles flexibility?

1. Attempt to stretch daily for around 10 minutes
2. Stretch until pain, since pain will mean you are getting a good stretch
3. You will gain the most flexibility by stretching as soon as you wake up as the tendon has relaxed the whole night
4. All of the above

(see page 139)

Strengthening Principles

Here are the basic rules I use for strengthening exercises. I always love to learn the exercises a physical therapist has shown my patients.

1. Begin to strengthen the day before an injury happens or the day before the patient sees you for the first time (thus, ASAP). This emphasizes the immediacy of begin strengthening.
2. Even though injuries have a definite period of Re-Strengthening, strengthening should begin immediately and continue well after the injury is finished completely healing.
3. Strengthen the injured area but also above and below the injured area. One of the best examples is patellofemoral syndrome where strengthening needs to be at the knee, but equally important at the hip and foot/ankle.
4. You should consider removable boot, ankle foot orthotic devices, foot orthotic devices, braces, and taping all part of the Immobilization Phase in an injury until the body gets strong enough to not need these devices. Of course, for many reasons, some assistive aid like orthotic devices may become permanent (at least for the most stressful activities like running) but that should not minimize the need to stay strong. For example, patients in stage II PTTD who are trying to avoid surgery may always be in orthotic devices or some other braces, while their daily strengthening program will keep all the anti-pronation muscles strong.
5. Since podiatrists deal with over pronation syndrome constantly, strengthening should consist of foot intrinsic muscles, posterior tibial tendon, anterior tibial tendon, peroneus longus tendon, gastrocnemius and soleus muscles, pes anserinus tendon group, lateral hamstring, and external hip rotators like gluteus minimus, gluteus medius, iliopsoas, and piriformis.
6. Since podiatrists deal with over supination syndrome constantly, strengthening should consist of both peroneal tendons, hip adductors, medial hamstrings while making sure the lateral hamstrings have normal flexibility, and internal hip rotators.

#80 When a patient is a severe pronator, which muscles are not helpful to strengthen?
1. Posterior Tibial Tendon

2. Internal Hip Rotators
3. Piriformis
4. Soleus
5. Peroneus Longus

(see page 139)

Helping with the Excessively Tight Tendons

There are 4 common techniques utilized by doctors and physical therapists when normal stretching is not helping. These are:
1. Mobilization of the Muscle Belly
2. Contract Relax Techniques
3. Various Splints
4. Prolonged Heat and Ice Constant Stretch

Mobilization of the muscle belly is a very important way of gaining flexibility when normal 3-5 times daily stretching is not enough. It normally needs a PT prescription of 4-8 visits. Measuring the flexibility beforehand yourself, sending the patient for 4 sessions, continuing them with their home program during the same period, and then re-measuring them is the best method to see if it will work. Contrast relax is a common stretching principle utilizing many by personal trainers, but my patients can be taught to do it with a partner. There are various methods of contract relax but I typically teach a 2 minute program. Let us use the hamstrings as an example. The patient is supine with their calf on their partner's shoulder and the hamstring being stretched for the entire 2 minutes. The patient then for a 6 second count contracts the hamstring by bending the knee against the partner's shoulder. The partner then stretches the hamstring more for 10 seconds,

and the contraction for 6 seconds begins again. This is repeated for 1-2 minutes or until any pain or cramping occurs. This is done at least 3 times a week. There are various splints that can be worn to gently stretch an area out while you are sleeping or at rest typing on your computer. You want to wear these splints at least 30 minutes at a time on a daily basis to gain. The DeHeer Equinus Brace for achilles tightness shows some good promise as it is the only achilles brace designed for the gastrocnemius. Finally, prolonged heat and ice stretches are effective (called Temple University Stretch). The heat application to the muscle belly is two times longer than the ice while the patient does continues to stretch. It is important not to have pain. It is crucial that the patient maintains the stretch as the heat is being replaced by ice. I have used this technique on achilles/calf tightness, quadriceps tightness, and hamstring tightness. I typically start at 10 minutes of heat and 5 minutes of ice, but have gone as high as 30 and 15. I typically do it first in the office so I can measure the before and after. The patient is told they can put on the hot pack to begin the process, but someone else needs to remove the heat and place on the ice since the stretch can not be broken. The heat and ice applications are for the muscle belly. This is typically done 2-3 times per week at home, and any time the patient is having physical therapy.

#81 Which of the following is not an adjunctive therapy for gaining flexibility?
1. Physical therapy mobilization

2. Braces for prolonged stretches
3. Contract Relax
4. Heat Ice where the heat is in equal amounts to the ice

(see page 139)

Appendix 8: 19 Common Foot Orthotic Cast Correction Prescription Variables

There are so many parts to a good custom made orthotic device that can be used to help a patient. I believe that the digital scanners are the future, but I still take neutral position suspension casts, since I have so many years experience and know what this cast gives me. I also feel that the research on the digital scanners is in its infancy and work needs to be done understanding it better. This book is about one aspect of orthotic devices, and not really a book on the complexity of orthotic devices with all its variables. However, the Inverted Orthotic Technique is about cast corrections, and this appendix is about the standard cast corrections I see in the industry, and cast correction is about what you are trying to change. I urge practitioners to look at how they are prescribing for pronators, neutral patients, and supinators and see how it correlates to this list. Are you practicing at your potential, or is there improvement that is possible? Most of the time, practitioners are limited to some extent by the expertise of the lab. I do not know how many of these techniques are made by individual labs, but each of these techniques are made by professional laboratories that I have been exposed to, and constantly exposed through patients whose orthotics are made by other practitioners. The following is a list of 19 cast corrections that can be utilized on any foot cast. There is also the plastic part and what you apply to the plastic part that makes for the very uniqueness of a custom orthotic device. Please do not forget that what you do for the right side may not be what you do for the left side. It is important to know that these are the standard corrections in the industry, with each lab offering several to 10 of them possibly. It is also important to know that the numbers assigned are pretty accurate in general within 2 degrees of change (so 8 degrees may be 6 up to 10 based on how the patient responds). I have also placed in bold the types I use most frequently day to day which I have the most reliable feel for what they give me in terms of body corrections. I am starting with the correction for the most supinated and ending with the most pronated.

Corrective Devices for Excessive Supination

Type A: 5 Degree Everted Orthotic Device with LCC, Feehery, and Lateral Kirby Skive

This is to place the heel vertical, but due to a tremendous inversion force at the heel, the cast correction must be loaded with equally tremendous eversion forces. It is so important to follow all the principles at stabilizing the lateral column in casting (complete maximally pronated casts since a supinated cast destabilizes the lateral column) and cast correction (like no fill in the cuboid area). Here is where it is important to remove any forefoot supinatus in the casting. Typically a slightly narrower orthotic device in general to de-emphasize the medial column is used. Typically you will also use 3/16th polypropylene, 25-28 mm lateral heel cups, lateral phalange, Denton modification, and may be forced into a ⅛ inch valgus wedge. The orthotic devices has a full length top cover and a forefoot valgus extension of ⅛ to ¼ inch utilized. If you use the ¼ inch forefoot extension, you want it 2nd to 5th metatarsal head. The ⅛ inch can be only under 4 and 5. Remember, for these first 3 orthotic devices listed, you are trying to make a supinator neutral not into a pronator. LCC stands for lateral column correction with minimal lateral arch fill, especially around the cuboid. LCC always implies to me that the lateral column is the most precious aspect of the correction from maximally pronated midtarsal joints in the cast, removing any supinatus possible, devaluing the medial presence in width and arch height and medial aspect of the rearfoot post.

Type B: 5 Degree Everted Orthotic Device with LCC

This is the same as A without the Lateral Kirby Skive and Feehery. You are just trying to develop a force to eliminate heel contact supination and its damaging forces, you are not trying to significantly pronate someone. Again, the importance of lateral column support can not be underestimated in

the casting technique, removing any forefoot supinatus, in the cast correction, and in the heel cups, phalanges, modifications, posts, and positive wedges. You can always put a temporary lateral Kirby or temporary Feehery at dispense.

Type C: Root Balanced Orthotic Device with Lower Medial Arch, Lateral Column Correction, and Lateral Kirby or Feehery

Emphasize the lateral arch grabbing the foot well. Typically made with a narrower cut medially (less medial support). This is a very common orthotic device. All the lateral stabilizing techniques may be used, although the cast is corrected to vertical. In dealing with a supination force at heel contact, you will want to remove any forefoot supinatus. It works so well in everted forefoot deformities. Lateral phalanges in general are crucial with any force that will produce transverse plane abduction of the forefoot on the rearfoot. I like the lateral Kirby when the lateral heel is flat to grab the lateral heel better, the lateral column correction with inverted forefoot deformities, and Feehery when there is ligamentous laxity so unstable cuboid.

Stabilizing Orthotic Device

Type D: Root Balanced Orthotic Device to Heel Vertical (Your Standard Orthotic)

This is the standard orthotic device that started modern day orthotic devices.

In order for practitioners to talk about biomechanical cases, you must be able tell how far from standard the orthotic device being used lies. This Root Balanced Orthotic Device supports all 3 arches equally captured in the impression cast. These are the medial, lateral, and metatarsal arches. The exact amount of forefoot varus or forefoot valgus is corrected. This is not a Modified Root Orthotic Device where the forefoot varus or valgus support is reduced, or the cast manipulated in some way. This is the balancing orthotic device of the forefoot to rearfoot relationship attained by an impression cast of the foot with the subtalar joint in neutral position and the midtarsal joint maximally pronated. I call this a stabilizing orthotic device as it gives incredible support and stability. When there is a lot of forefoot valgus, sometimes due to a plantar flexed first ray, it is a truly corrective orthotic device for excessive supination or pronation. This is the orthotic construction every orthotic laboratory should know how to make, and know when they are modifying away from and why (comfort, allowing more support in any one arch over another, allowing for more forward motion, etc). I prefer to make all of my soft based orthotics, except the Hannafords, from a Root Balanced mold.

Corrective Devices for Abnormal Pronation

Type E: D plus MMS meaning maximal metatarsal support

Small, but powerful, change when you have metatarsal problems and you need more support for bunions, neuromas, metatarsalgia, hammertoes, etc. In my mind, the support of the metatarsals is the weakest link in a custom orthotic device, as the impression cast only truly captures the skin. Many patients then need over the counter metatarsal pads to fill in the gap between orthotic and metatarsals. MMS allows the lab to add around 1/16th inch plastic under those metatarsals, yet it is still common to need more soft metatarsal pads to be typically placed under the metatarsal arch on the plastic and sandwiched under the top cover. For many patients, it is the metatarsal support that is the most important of the 3 arches, and there are also those patients where the medial and lateral arches are the most important arch to support. Sometimes, it is not easy to predict.

Type F: D plus MCC meaning medial column correction

Here you are telling the laboratory to give you the highest arch they can (although still continue the peak of support under the navicular 1st cuneiform joint, and sometimes they will hardly put any fill on the mold so that when you press the plastic the medial arch will come out high. Dr. Paul Scherer, from ProLab USA, advocated that this higher arch position was being captured in every impression cast taken by slightly plantarflexing the first metatarsal while you casted the foot. I use MCC commonly in the Inverted Technique staging where I am going to make a higher new orthotic device for more correction (probably just one degree more support or 5-10% more support) or an initial Inverted Orthotic Device in pes cavus patients when they do not have lateral instability. Instead of putting in more inversion, like going from a 25 to 35 degree correction, I simply add an MCC and medial Kirby to the present mold giving approximately 3 more degrees of correction. This probably should be standard with pes cavus foot type in the industry as long as the lateral column is protected. When you are utilizing soft based orthotic devices, the LEO cast correction from Burns Laboratory (lateral expansion only) can make a great device without concern for blocking first metatarsal plantarflexion yet capturing the high arch. For heel pain, it is a wonderful modification to transfer weight from the heel to the arch. Unless you are using a lot of rear foot inversion (30 or 35 degrees inversion) for forefoot abduction problems, this is the second best method at preventing the foot from abducting laterally off the orthotic device. Even though there is no inversion with the Type F: Root Balanced with MCC, clinically you see about a one degree change towards less pronation.

Type G: 15 Degrees Inverted Orthotic Technique with LCC (lateral column correction) and Lateral Kirby Skives

This is the classic technique for medial and lateral instability patients. The 15 degrees of the Inverted Orthotic Technique will give you 3 degrees of inversion (5 to 1 ratio of cast corrections to actual inversion force to the foot with the Inverted Technique).

With this technique, you are basically trying to place equal forces of inversion and eversion, to hold the foot vertical. Even though not that commonly utilized, I have tried to balance the forces with a similar Root Balanced technique in three ways for this medial and lateral instability foot:

1. Root Balanced with forefoot valgus support when present and medial Kirby skive
2. Root Balanced with Feehery cuboid or LCC and high lateral heel cups and lateral phalanges with medial Kirby skive
3. Root Balanced Technique with MCC and lateral Kirby skive and high medial and lateral heel cups (25-28 mm)

Type H: D plus Medial Kirby Skive or F plus Medial Kirby Skive

The medial skive was designed by Dr. Kevin Kirby of Sacramento, California as a way of supporting the medial side of the subtalar joint to help with pronation control. His excellent paper on subtalar joint axis evaluation is a must read in foot biomechanics. The medial Kirby Skive is used here to give 2 degrees more varus support to the rearfoot which would be equivalent to 10 degrees inverted pour with the Inverted Orthotic Technique. If the Kirby skive, Root Balance, and Medial Column Correction are utilized together, then 3 degrees of varus support are typically achieved which is equivalent to a 15 degree correction with the Inverted Orthotic Technique.

Type I: 15 Degree Inverted Orthotic Technique

Standard starting correction for the Inverted Orthotic Technique. This gives 3 degrees of pronation support. Used when the pronation is considered mild, but symptomatic, and knee alignment may also be important in bringing a slight heel valgus to vertical, or a vertical heel in resting to inverted position for tibial varum alignment. This is used in patients where there is medial and lateral instability (see Type G). These are patients that you could classify as pronators and supinators. For example someone that walks or runs with pronation type symptoms, but has had many lateral ankle sprains in the past and you do not want to risk more sprains.

Type J: 25 Degree Inverted Orthotic Technique

This is my default anti-pronation orthotic device with its 5 degrees of pronation support for moderate to severe pronators. When I watch a patient walk or run, and they are a pronator, I try to imagine what this Type J orthotic device will give me, or do I need more varus support or less varus support with more lateral column support. This is my classic runner's orthotic device, like the 4-6 degree runner's wedges I made

as a student under the great supervision of Drs. Steven Subotnick, Ronald Valmassy, Richard Bogdan, and Harry Hlavac.

Type K: 5 Degree Inverted Pour with MCC

This is different than the Inverted Technique since it is a straight inversion of the cast. Commonly done for when the resting heel position is vertical, but the neutral subtalar joint position is inverted from tibial varum. With the MCC, you will get 6 or so degrees of varus support. Typically, this is your classic runner's wedge in an orthotic device for running limb varus conditions when you are not utilizing the Inverted Technique. I first saw this with many patients using KLM labs in Los Angeles, California, from orthotic devices that my podiatry partner Dr. William Olson made. KLM was also his chief investigators for the new carbon graphite TL61 that he had invented. Typically used in forefoot valgus feet. You would have to use a Modified Root with neutral forefoot or forefoot varus feet (due to the abrupt first metatarsal modifications needed in these feet, severe deviations from classic Root buildup).

Type L: 15 Degree Inverted Pour with MCC and Medial Kirby

This is a very popular Inverted Orthotic Device that is technically easy for the labs, and their scanners, to accomplish. When I am dealing with orthotic labs in general, they typically feel more comfortable placing less inversion in the cast correction, but that varies tremendously. They have a point, that I will discuss, that the higher inversions from my technique can lead to some loss of the original foot perspective (reference points) by the technician. You accomplish 3 degrees of correction with the Inversion, 2 degrees with the Medial Kirby, and another degree with the MCC totalling 6 degrees. With a patient standing 6-8 degrees everted, you can expect to help their alignment get close to a vertical heel positioning.

Type M: 35 Degree Inverted Orthotic Technique

This is my highest initial (starting point) inversion for the severe pronators in walking or running, even if I estimate they will need more later (I restrict the initial correction due to the breakin adjustments expected with such a high change). Typically 7 degrees on average will be changed in the resting position, so that a severely everted heel of 7-8 degrees can be expected to be placed close to vertical. In cases where the heel position is everted, vertical, or inverted with rearfoot varus (like high tibial varum), you can change the heel position to a more inverted heel position of 4-7 degrees.
If we take a patient with collapsed arches with 13 degrees everted resting position, for example, the 35 degrees will give them a great correction going in the right direction. 3-4 months later, the molds can be adjusted higher, once they are used to the change. Just prior to this writing my last patient was typical change from 14 everted to 10 everted with a 35 degree correction. He had 22 degrees of forefoot varus/supinatus in the

cast. This is badly pronated foot. But, the next more minor reset typically will give more degrees of correction than expected.

Type N: 25 Degree Inverted Pour with MCC and Medial Kirby

This gives about 8 degrees change for pronation support. Labs and scanners like dealing with less inversion if you can get similar results. I like MCC, or less arch fill, particularly in pes cavus feet, which in general never get enough medial arch support. Patients with pes cavus that get good arch support for the first time are my happiest orthotic patients. Remember, MCC should remain a proximal support (only to the 1st cuneiform base) so as to not block the first ray plantarflexion.

Type O: 5 Degree Inverted Pour with MCC and Medial Kirby

Again different than the Inverted Orthotic Technique since it is a straight inversion so you have to be concerned with the anterior platform transition to not block first ray plantarflexion. Technique works ideally best in everted forefoot deformities (forefoot valgus or plantarflexed first ray) so that the medial transition at the anterior platform will not block first ray plantarflexion. Typically gives 8 degrees of varus correction, so perfect as a running orthotic device for Running Limb Varus. Please consider separating your running devices from your walking devices when you use inversion forces like Type O.

With the great Dual Density Midsole running shoes out there have for pronation support, these varus corrections are used, but now less frequently. Again, typically used in forefoot valgus feet, or with a Modified Root in neutral or forefoot varus feet (in order to smooth the transition at the distal medial corner of the orthotic device and not block first metatarsal plantar flexion for push off). However, this is one of the reasons Dr. Root supported my technique originally since the proximal support could be clearly differentiated from classic Root device. Once we start using a variety of modified Root devices, which typically lose some support of the medial, metatarsal, and lateral columns, some of the science of orthotic devices goes out the window. Research is needed on these modified Root corrections.

Type P: 8 Degrees Inverted Pour with MCC (typically not forefoot varus feet)

Different from the Inverted Orthotic Technique since it is straight inversion. Any forefoot varus is ignored (meaning that the plaster from the medial arch is smoothed into the platform). This is a modified Root device, except when patient has 8 or more degrees of everted forefoot deformity (forefoot valgus, forefoot pronatus, or plantar flexed first ray). It will typically give you 8-10 degrees of inversion, used for exclusively as a running orthotic device (at least what I have seen), or PTTD patients.

Type Q: 35 Degree Inverted Technique with MCC and Medial Kirby

This is typically the second highest correction, as I have found higher inversion distorts from the original foot too much on a consistent basis. In these severe pronators, this is usually a simple repress to the initial orthotic device set at 35 degrees Inverted in which I have now added a medial Kirby and MCC up to the 1st cuneiform base. This allows 10 degrees of pronation support. If coupled with stable shoes, ¼ inch varus midsole shoe wedging, power lacing, you can easily get up to 14 degrees of correction. When I measure a relaxed heel position over 10 degrees everted, I will use the straight 35 degree correction initially, get the patient used to it, and then take the same mold and add the medial Kirby and MCC prior to repressing the orthotic device. In my practice I only see 20 patients per year needing more correction then this. With these severely pronated feet that you are controlling to such a degree, it is important after impression casting to measure the forefoot to rearfoot angle captured in the cast. As you follow them, it may be good to recast them at least one year later to see if the cast captured less supinatus. You may be able to make a better orthotic device off the new cast for them at that point. I want to see all of these patients yearly for this purpose.

Type R: 10 Degrees Inverted Pour with MCC and Medial Kirby

Highest corrected standard modified Root orthotic device on the market that I have seen. Used in forefoot varus feet over 10 degrees (since classic Root support would block first ray plantarflexion). Gives 10-13 degrees of pronation support. Ideal as a running orthotic also due to the severe pronation in some runners at heel strike.

Type S: 45 Degree Inverted Reset of Type Q

The highest angle I use on patients and it is always a reset to the original mold. Type Q is transitioned to this product already having a medial Kirby and MCC (medial column correction). To protect the lateral column further, I have the laboratory put the new anterior platform on top of the old 35 degree inverted platform. This actually allows me to place a slight lateral arch transition from platform to 5th metatarsal shaft. I have to make sure I rework the lateral expansion to be parallel to the new platform. I make sure the new medial expansion covers proximally to the 1st cuneiform only. I make sure I carefully watch the lateral column to be parallel to the new platform, and the two lateral contact points are 5th metatarsal head area and lateral heel. If the contact point drifts out onto the midfoot, the Feehery technique or simply lateral column correction has to elevate the midfoot. This is an extremely powerful device which already has the medial modifications, so that the average pronator responds 12 degrees. When you add shoes, lacing, midsole wedges, taping if needed, etc, over 20 degrees of change can be produced. This has been tested over and over again.

In Summary:
This is the highest correction I use in a functional foot orthotic device. This correction changes the foot 12 degrees on average. The mold has been already set at 35 degrees Inverted with Medial Kirby and Medial Column Correction. I do not remove the original platform set at 35, I add another platform on top of that to get 2 more degrees of inversion correction, while continuing to protect the lateral column. I have found this method to dramatically lessen the distortion of the foot to the cast. You have to make sure the lateral column in releveled parallel to the new anterior platform. You may have to adjust the medial Kirby and medial column correction for smoothness and make sure the peak of the medial arch remains under the navicular first cuneiform and does not drift anterior to that.

Occasionally, when you heavily invert someone, and significantly raise the adult acquired flat foot, the patient's heel will look better, but they will hang up in the arch and the first metatarsal can not get to the ground. In these cases, you need to build a platform distally to support the medial column. This may change over time, with a lessening of the support needed, but you need to maintain good medial column stability with a forefoot extension that starts around the base of the first metatarsal. The images below should give you an idea of this support needed. Physical therapy to mobilize the tissues can also help with particularly sagittal and frontal plane contractures.

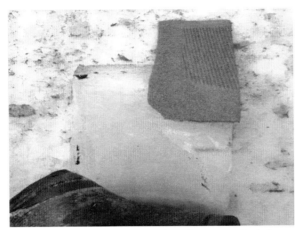

Here the forefoot extension is extended from the first metatarsal base to the base of the hallux

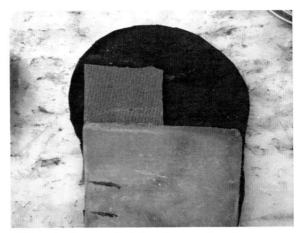

Here is the medial forefoot extension seen from plantarly. Goal is to load the first metatarsal to the supporting surface for stability. These forefoot extensions can just be extended Morton's extensions to very supportive 1st through 4th metatarsal varus skives.

#82 When utilizing the Inverted Orthotic Technique, what is the highest inversion that is used as a starting point?
1. 25 Degrees
2. 35 Degrees
3. 45 Degrees
4. None of these

(see page 139)

#83 When utilizing the Inverted Orthotic Technique, what is the modification called when the forefoot valgus is also captured in the positive correction?
1. Denton Modification
2. Feehery Modification
3. Fettig Modification
4. Kirby Modification
5. Valmassy Modification

(see page 139)

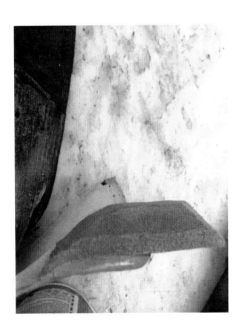

This is the view of the forefoot extension from the medial side

#84 With severely pronated feet, the utilization of the Inverted Orthotic Technique can potentially produce how many degrees of less pronation change when combined with other modalities?

1. 7 degrees
2. 10 degrees
3. 15 degrees
4. 20 degrees

(see page 139)

#85 When utilizing the Inverted Technique to gain degrees of pronation correction, name 3 of the common modifications that will gain 1 to 2 degrees more support routinely:

1. _____
2. _____
3. _____

(see page 139)

#86 Which degrees of the Inverted Orthotic Technique is considered the default degrees to base all correction?

1. 10
2. 15
3. 20
4. 25
5. 30
6. 35

(see page 139)

#87 Typical patient with 10 degrees of forefoot varus, 5 degrees of tibial varum, will have the resting heel position at 5 degrees everted. Does the following correction help this patient with posterior tibial tendon pain? (Yes or No) 3 degrees of forefoot varus in cast correction, and 2 degrees gained by medial Kirby Skive.

(see page 139)

Appendix 9: Impression Cast Technique and Comments on Digital Scanning

https://youtu.be/T81AJEVPEQI

The neutral suspension cast where the subtalar joint is placed in neutral position and the midtarsal joints are held maximally pronated is the gold standard for the orthotic device industry. The cast replicates the most stable position of the foot capturing the forefoot to rearfoot deformity. Plaster of Paris splints are utilized to make such a cast, and three splints are applied to the foot, the joints are placed in their ideal positions, and then the splints are rubbed in with good pressure with one hand while the other hand keeps the joint positions and the anterior tibial tendon relaxed. It is the cast I always try to make perfect. I do not want any experimentation here. The cast has to be the same today as it was 25 years ago, or I can not see how the foot has changed. You should be able to take the same cast as I can on the same patient if we have similar training (all podiatry schools teach this technique of neutral suspension casting). I encourage you to contact Jeff Root at info@root-lab.com for information on casting. I have the 1971 Neutral Casting Book by Drs. Root, Weed, and Orien, but I am sure it is out of print. In every area there is a podiatrist known for their orthotic casting. Try to see if they will give a workshop. If you and I can take the same cast, and if I ask for 3 degrees of inversion, and you ask the lab to put in 4 degrees, the two orthotic devices made should reflect that. This is the ideal, and what we should shoot for as a profession with the teaching in our schools.

More of the reality lies in my own use of the cast in my lifetime as a podiatrist. Podiatrists tend, and I think this is overall good practice, to take their impression casts the way that they think best, and then fill out a prescription sheet for an orthotic lab that does all of their business. They get comfortable with the orthotic lab and know what to expect from the lab. This relationship is at the heart of podiatry. Most functional orthotic devices I see from other podiatrists are good or great. Most orthotic devices I make for my patients are good or great. But, maybe what I think is great, 20 years from now will be fair to poor. How do we (as individuals, as a profession, and as the orthotic laboratory industry) get better?

These are the steps for the next 20 years that I think should happen based on my knowledge that the Root Neutral Suspension Cast is the ideal method of capturing foot structure. It is the only cast technique I would have my sons or grandson casted with. I have seen every cast technique out there and the Root Neutral Suspension Cast Technique gives the most functional orthotic device. The steps are:

1. Orthotic Laboratories should put on workshops for casting and/or proper digital scanning.
2. The Podiatry Colleges should put on workshops for casting and/or digital scanning.
3. There should be research published for the practicing podiatrist on the difference in these 2 venues, Root suspension casting versus digital scanning.
4. The differences in foam box impression casting versus suspension casting should be analyzed, or other popular methods.

To this day, billions of orthotic devices have been made off suspension casts with relatively great results. I feel that way, and I have never seen a research paper doubt its abilities to accurately capture the foot. In the future, it is more what the podiatrist does with the cast, then the cast itself, that can change the foot function. Even if the cast accuracy and reproducibility is vital to my practice, the Inverted Orthotic Technique basically makes a new foot with cast corrections.

I usually make all my orthotic devices, along with the manufacturing help of my brother Robert Blake, and I know exactly what I am going to get for the prescription I am using. I tried to do a small experiment where I digitally casted 5 patients and emailed the impression and prescription to the laboratory. I then casted each patient and made the orthotic devices in the traditional way. These 2 orthotics were so much different, and I do not live close to the laboratory I used, that I shut down the experiment. The patients may have even liked the digital scanned ones the best in some cases, but I shut the experiment down since I did not know what I was getting. This bothered me greatly. I also once tried to play craps, and on the first roll of the dice when they took the money I placed down, and I had no clue why they took my money, I walked away from the table. Predictability is crucial with orthotic devices. This is why many doctors have developed their comfort zone with orthotic devices and will not vary. I believe that the Inverted Orthotic Technique is worth coming out of your comfort zone for the health of your patients.

I recently chatted with Jeff Root, from Root Functional Orthotic Laboratory, and he is very happy with the digital scanning results. Even when you send a negative impression cast into the laboratory, they will digital scan the cast and start the CAD-CAM process. I think overall the future is bright with this technology. But, you still need to know how to hold the foot the correct way even with the digital scanners.

#88 Digital scanners should be able to accurately capture the foot as well or better than an impression cast? _____
(see page 139)

Appendix 10: Advice for Adjustment to the Inverted Orthotic Technique

Patient Handout

Breaking into full time wear of custom made functional foot orthotic devices should occur over a period of 10 to 14 days, and it is even more important in the Inverted Orthotic Technique. You are making changes to the entire body and it is important to gradually add more stress.

On the day you pick up the orthotic devices, wear them for 1 hour if tolerated. This hour should only include active walking or standing. Do not count sitting time. Therefore, 1 hour of orthotic wear may actually occur over 2 to 6 hours of real time. If even 1 hour is difficult, attempt (2) 30 minute sessions, or (4) 15 minute sessions, with an hour off between sessions.

The breaking in process continues by adding 1 more hour each day until you are up to 8 hours by the 8th day. Of course, due to many factors, it may take more than 8 days to build up to 8 hours, and you may never stand or walk for 8 hours per day unless you go on vacation. You may not even walk or stand 8 hours in any given day on average. Once you are at 8 hours, you should be able to go as long as you desire on any given day. Runners should run 1 mile longer with the orthotic devices each day (starting at 1 mile on the first day). You should finish your normal distance with your old orthotic devices or the shoe inserts. Depending on how much change in your biomechanics has been prescribed, at times your doctor will recommend that you get used to them for a week before wearing them in the stressful situations of your

sporting activity. Other athletic activities, especially side to side sports like basketball, should progress in 30 minute intervals daily (starting with 30 minutes the first day). It is never a good idea to get used to new orthotic devices, even brand new shoes, while you are ramping up your mileage like when training for a marathon.

If you get discomfort anywhere (foot, ankle, knee, hip, or back) while breaking in the device, immediately remove the device, and leave it out of your shoe for the next 2 hours. If there is still time later in the day, you can try to re-wear them if you have not met your time allotment.

It is important during the adjustment period to always have the regular shoe inserts (or your old orthotics) with you in case you have to take out your orthotic devices for this 2 hour period. The accommodation period is partially for foot comfort, but mainly for the knee, hip, and back adjustment to the new positioning of the body and the new use of many muscle groups.

Golden Rule: Always blame any new ache or pain on the new orthotic devices. Never push through any pain, no matter how insignificant it seems. The breaking in process must be pain free.

Normally patients are told to get used to their orthotic devices and return in 6 weeks. However, 30% of patients return to the office in 2 weeks or so since they are having some troubles with their orthotic devices, and can not wear the orthotics more than several hours.

Adjustments are normally routine and part of normal office visits. Occasionally the orthotic devices or impression molds must be returned to the laboratory for further fine-tuning.

The doctor/therapist prescribing the orthotic devices should dispense them, watch you walk and or run, and attempt to make the devices more stable and comfortable if appropriate. This is the perfect time to learn power lacing, if it works with the shoes you have. Power lacing, also called stability knot and runner's knot, is a must for orthotic devices as it prevents heel slippage and greatly adds to stability.

The prescribing practitioner may use their judgement when allowing some discomfort or uncomfortable pressure, if further adjustments could lead to loss of stability. This is a fine line because the inserts must be comfortable enough to have you want to wear them. Wear socks with the inserts when there is no smooth top cover. Some practitioners only dispense a purely plastic device.

If the devices squeak with certain shoes, remove the orthotic device from the shoe and apply powder (any type, although corn starch may lead to infections) to the inside of the shoe. Rub the powder along the sides of the inner liner where the orthotic device will be in contact with the shoe. This normally takes care of the squeaking for several months. Some of our patients have used body glide or slip hose (thin nylon) over the orthotic devices which accomplish the same function. In the office, your prescribing practitioner can place leather or

suede over the parts of the orthotic device causing the noise.

When the orthotic device has a top cover, occasionally noise is produced by an air pocket developing under the heel. Carefully pull up the top cover if possible in the heel area. This can be reglued down at your next visit, or Superglue can help tack it back down.

When you are given orthotic devices with top covers, it is helpful to check the device bimonthly to reattach any loose sections with Superglue. The practitioner may not tightly attach the top cover initially if multiple adjustments for improved comfort and stability are anticipated.

If the shoe utilized has a removable insert, and that insert has definite firm structure, remove it completely. You want the orthotic device to sit down in the shoe as low as possible for stability. However, if you need more padding, apply a thin flat insert to the front or full length under the orthotic device. These are commonly found in Dr. Scholls or Spenco product lines. You can usually cut out the heel section of this added layer leaving the rest of the insert. This allows the orthotic device to drop as low as possible into the shoe. Hopefully the prescribing doctor has made sure the orthotic device itself sits down in the shoe completely.

When receiving small dress orthotic devices, you need some short insoles for the front of the shoe (unless it is attached as an extension to your orthosis) in order to hold your foot from slipping out of the heel in some shoes. The orthotic device should not be wider than the shoe because this pushes the shoe away from your foot.

Dress orthotic devices normally require little time to get used to so breaking into them should be quick. However, listen to your body and remove the orthotic device for two hours if you have any new discomfort anywhere in your body. If you find that you need to grip with your toes in order to hold the shoes on with the inserts, more front padding must be used. Dr. Scholls does sell this product. There are some shoes that will not work with your new inserts for this reason. Unfortunately, you may need to take the orthotic devices with you to buy some new shoes, since the original shoes were not fitted with orthotic devices in mind.

Some corrective orthotic devices, like the Inverted Orthotic Technique, follow most of these rules but have other issues discussed by your practitioner if they occur. Also, the memory foam orthotic devices Hannaford style take 30 hours of wear to compress 30% before they are a good fit in your shoe. Explain to your provider what you are experiencing at all times so they can tell if something needs adjustment, or just further adjustment time by you. Good Luck and we hope the mechanical change produced is very healthy for your body.

#89 If the patient received new orthotic devices, especially highly corrective Inverted Orthotic Devices, and pain is experienced, what is the best treatment?

1. Take out the new orthotic devices from your shoes and give your feet a week rest.
2. Ignore the pain since it is a common experience as you adjust to the inserts.
3. If you begin to get some new knee symptoms, it has nothing to do with the new inserts, since there is no relationship of the foot to the knee.
4. None of the above

(see page 139)

Appendix 11: References for the Inverted Orthotic Technique

The following are the previous articles published on the Inverted Orthotic Technique.

- Inverted Functional Orthosis. Blake RL. J. Am. Podiatr Med Assoc. 1986 May;76(5): 275-6.
- Foot Orthosis for Severe Flatfoot in Sports. Blake RL, Ferguson HA. J. Am. Podiatr Med Assoc. 1991 Oct; 81(10): 549-55
- Biomechanical analysis of Running with 25 degree inverted orthotic devices. Baitch SP, Blake RL, Fineagan PL, Senatore J. J. Am. Podiatr Med Assoc. 1991 Dec; 81(12): 647-52.
- The Inverted Orthotic Technique: A practical discussion of an orthotic therapy. Blake RL. J.Brit.Pod. Med. Feb 1993; 48(2).
- Update and Rationale for the Inverted Functional Foot Orthosis. Blake, RL. Clinics in Podiatric Med and Surg. April 1994; 11(2).
- The Inverted Orthotic Technique: Its Role in Clinical Biomechanics. Blake RL, Ferguson HA. Clinical Biomechanics of the Lower Extremities, Dr. Ronald Valmassy, editor, Mosby YearBook, Inc. 1995; Chapter 22: pages 466-497.
- Effect of inverted orthoses on lower extremity mechanics for runners. Williams DS 3rd, McClay Davis I, Baitch SP. Med Sci Sports Exerc. 2003 Dec; 35(12): 260-8.
- Effect of foot orthotics on rearfoot and tibial joint coupling patterns and variability. Ferber R, Davis IM, Williams DS 3rd. J. Biomechanics. 2005 Mar; 38(3): 477-83.
- Effect of foot posture and inverted foot orthoses on hallux dorsiflexion. Munteanu SE, Bassad AD. J. Am. Podiatr Med Assoc. 2006 Jan-Feb; 96(1): 32-7.
- The effect of three levels of foot orthotic wedging on the surface electromyographic activity of selective lower limb muscles in gait. Murley GS, Bird AR. Clin Biomech (Bristol, Avon). 2006 Dec; 21(10): 1074-80.
- Effects of Custom-Made Rigid Foot Orthosis on Pes Planus in Children over 6 Years Old. Bok SK, Kim BO, Lim JH, Ahn SY. Ann Rehabil Med. 2014 Jun; 38(3): 369-75.
- Effect of Foot Orthoses on Children with Lower Extremity Growing Pains. Lee HJ, Lim KB, Yoo J, Yoon SW, Jeong TH. Ann Rehabil Med. 2015 Apr; 39(2): 285-93.
- Adults with Flexible Pes Planus and the approach to the prescription of customized foot orthoses in clinical practice: A clinical records audit. Banwell HA, Thewlis D, Mackintosh S. Foot (Edinb). 2015 Jun; 25(2): 101-9.
- Effect of Custom-Molded Foot Orthoses on Foot Pain and Balance in Children With Symptomatic Flexible Flat Feet. Lee HJ, Lim KB, Yoo J, Yoon SW, Yun HJ, Jeong

TH. Ann Rehabil Med. 2015 Dec; 39(6): 905-13.

- The Effect of Different Foot Orthosis Inverted Angles on Plantar Pressures in Children with Flexible Flat Feet. Bok SK, Lee H, Kim BO, Ahn S, Song Y, Park I. PLoS One. 2016 Jul 26; 11(7).

- The Effects of Talus Control Foot Orthoses in Children with Flexible Flatfoot. Ahn SY, Bok SK, Kim BO, Park IS. J. Am. Podiatr Med Assoc. 2017 Jan; 107 (1): 46-53.

- Custom-made foot orthoses: an analysis of prescription characteristics from an Australian commercial orthotic laboratory. Menz HB, Allan JJ, Bonanno DR, Landorf KB, Murley GS. J. Foot Ankle Res. 2017 June 7; 10(23).

- The effectiveness of non-surgical intervention (Foot Orthoses) for paediatric flexible pes planus: A systematic review: Update. Dars S, Uden H, Banwell HA, Kumar S. PLoS One. 2018 Feb 16; 13(2).

- Long-Term Effect of Rigid Foot Orthosis in Children Older Than Six With Flexible Flat Feet. Youn KJ, Ahn SY, Kim BO, Park IS, Bok SK. Ann Rehabil Med. 2019 Apr; 43(2): 224-229.

Appendix 12: Answers to Self Test Questions for the Inverted Orthotic Technique

Answers to the Questions in this book on the Inverted Orthotic Technique

.

#1   9 all of the above (you can see how many avenues or modalities we have to help fight the pronation forces causing problems)

#2   7 (all of the above)

#3   1 (moderate to severe pronation)

#4   4 (forefoot varus poured as is)

#5   4 (Feehery is for the lateral arch)

#6   8 (all of the above)

#7   7 (all of the above)

#8   3 (least likely)

#9   5 (unlikely to vary shoes)

#10 5 (all of the above)

#11 5 (1 and 3 are not correct)

#12 3 (Neutral Shoes)

#13 5 (all of the above, 1 the best)

#14 6 (all of the above)

#15 7 (PT and Soleus)

#16 6 (3 and 4 correct)

#17 3 (example forefoot valgus only)

#18 5 (all of the above)

#19 Inverted with pronation
     Root Balanced with supination
     Hannaford with shock absorption
     Lifts for short leg syndrome

#20 3 related to genu recurvatum forces

#21 15 (all of the above)

#22 1 (flat post makes more rigid)

#23 3 (correction for Rearfoot Varus)

#24 6 (all of the above)

#25 5 (all of the above)

#26 1 (I am not a fan of pre-fabs)

#27 5 (history and gait should point you)

#28 3 Neutral (the rest of the names are non accurate)

#29 6 all of the above

#30 7 all of the above

#31 2 (hourly increases in walking or standing only)

#32 5 (all of the above)

#33 2 (pronation causes an anterior movement across the lateral femoral epicondyle)

#34 3 (the everted heel from forefoot varus compensation can produce valgus knee motion and lateral joint compression)

#35 2,4,5

#36 6 (both 2 and 4)

#37 4 (heel lift all weight on PF insertion)

#38 6 (both 2 and 4)

#39 4 (medial not lateral knee compartment compression with supination)

#40 4 (all of the above)

#41 5 (all of the above)

#42 6 (all of the above)

#43 5 (all of the above)

#44 5 (all of the above)

#45 6 (none of the above)

#46 Theraband (Phase 2)
     Prednisone (Phase 1)
     Cam Walker (Phase 1)
     Walk Run (Phase 3)
     4 Days Icing (Phase 1)
     Active ROM (Phase 1)

#47 Ankle Sprains and Forefoot Varus

#48 3 (0-2 pain levels)

#49 Mechanical, Inflammatory, and Neuropathic

#50 4 and 5

#51 7 (all of the above)

#52 3 (typically longer side pronates more)

#53 5 (normal pronation can put the heel temporarily everted)

#54 4 tibial stress fractures

#55 1 (push off through 1 and 2)

#56 2 Sinus Tarsi pain is typically pronatory

#57 4 (pes cavus is unpredictable and can pronate, supinate, or have relatively no motion at heel contact)

#58 5 (limb dominance can be from multiple problems)

#59 2 Forefoot varus (all other choices listed can produce heel inversion at heel contact)

#60 8 (all of the above)

#61 Lateral Instability with Peroneal
Internal Knee with Ext Hip Rotator
Arch Collapse with Post Tibial
Lack Heel Lift with Achilles
Lateral Lean with Hip Abductor

#62 1 (if they limp, you can not perform a good gait evaluation)

#63 4 (weak peroneus brevis)

#64 7 (all of the above)

#65 1, 2, 3

#66 6 (all of the above)

#67 4 (all of the above)

#68 1. Pronatory
2. No symptoms, unless pronatory due high tibial varum
3. Supinatory
4. No symptoms, unless over 3-4 degrees tibial varum

#69 3 Tibial Varum Deformity

#70 No, that would probably block first metatarsal plantarflexion for a great push off

#71 Jack's Test

#72 Gastrocnemius

#73 25 Degrees Inverted

#74 Morton's Extension

#75 NCSP 3 Inverted

#76 Sagittal

#77 3 (internal hip rotators are pronators)

#78 8 (all of the above)

#79 4 (all of the above)

#80 2 (Internal Hip Rotators)

#81 4 (heat should be twice the ice in duration)

#82 2 (35 Degrees Inverted)

#83 3 (Fettig Modification)

#84 4 (20 degrees)

#85 10 degree reset to more inversion, medial kirby skive, medial column correction, varus midsole wedging, changing to motion control shoe like Brooks Beast or Ariel

#86 4 (25 degrees)

#87 Yes, 5 degrees of support are gained to get the patient close to vertical. With cases like this, you need to follow the patient, and if the posterior tibial pain is not quick to resolve, especially with the tibial varum, you may have to get more inversion force at the heel with the Inverted Technique.

#88 Yes (I definitely want to see what the differences are, even how modifications to the classic Root devices are made from manual plaster work (like Kirby, Feehery, Inverted Technique, etc.)

#89 4 (none of the above)

Index

3 Approaches to Utilization of the Inverted Orthotic Technique 28-29
5 to 1 Relationship Inverted Cast Correction 8
12 Point Biomechanical Outline 65-67
19 Common Foot Orthotic Cast Correction Prescription Variables 121-30
25 Degree Inverted Orthotic Device 125
35 Degree Inverted Orthotic Device 126
45 Degree Inverted Orthotic Device 128

A

Achilles Strain 53
Achilles Strength 104
Actin and Myosin Filaments 104
Adjustments to Orthosis 13, 133-135
Adult Acquired Flat Feet 23, 26
Allied OSI Labs 5
Ambulator Extra Depth Shoe 101
Ankle Impingement 53, 60
Ankle Joint Dorsiflexion Non Weight Bearing 102-105
Ankle Joint Dorsiflexion Weight Bearing 105
Ankle Strength Testing 113-114
Answers to Self Test Questions 138-139
Anterior Cruciate Ligament 55
Anterior Platform 46-48
Anterior Tibial Tendonitis 53
Anterior Tibial Tendon Strength 113
Apropulsive Gait 78
Arch Height Determination 45
Asymmetry in Gait 10-11, 66

B

Basic Premise of the Inverted Orthotic Technique 23
Bi-axial or Tri-axial Orthosis 4
Biomechanical Causes of Injuries 4
Biomechanical Examination 85-86
Biomechanical Examination Basic Components 86-114
Biomechanical Patient Definition 31
Blog Information 3
Bowlegs 20, 111
Bouncy Gait 76
Break In Orthotic Advice 44, 133-135
Bunion Conservative Treatments 27, 52
Burns Podiatric Laboratory 17, 124

C

Categorizing Patient's Biomechanics 4, 31
Causes of Injury 31
Causes of Over Pronation 32-33
Checklist for Biomechanical Visit 65-66
Checklist for Gait Evaluation 69
Checklist for Pronation Produced Problems 56
Checklist for Supination Produced Problems 63
Checklist of Available Modalities to Help with Pronation 117
Children 40-41
Collapsed Arch 78-79
Conclusion 51
Contact Phase and the Inverted Orthotic Device 16
Contact Phase Lateral Instability 80
Contract Relax Stretching 120
Corrective Orthotic Devices for Pronators 123-129

Corrective Orthotic Devices for Supinators 121-122

Correction over 35 Degrees 37-38

Correction Proves Too Little 36-39

Correction Proves Too Much 34-35

Correction Requirements for Orthotic Devices 27

Cross Training Biomechanically 42

Cuboid Syndrome 53, 59

Customizing OTC inserts 33

D

Dancer's Padding 26, 100

DeHeer Equinus Brace 120

Denton Modification 13, 19-20, 29, 34-35, 112, 122

Determining the Arch Height 45

Differential Diagnosis 65

Digital Scanning 132

Dominance in Gait 80

Double Crush Syndrome 25

Dr. Richard Bogdan 17, 125

Dr. Joseph D'Amico 3

Dr. Howard Dannenberg 3, 16, 99

Dr. Jane Denton 6

Dr. Raymond Feehery 5, 19

Dr. Mathias Fettig 5, 19

Dr. Harry Hlavac 17, 125

Dr. Kevin Kirby 3, 112, 124

Dr. Sheldon Langer 3

Dr. Ross Leonard 25

Dr. Richard Lundeen 5

Dr. Merton Root 3, 16, 18, 24-25, 27, 76, 77, 89, 99, 110, 127, 130

Dr. William Olson 5, 125

Dr. William Orien 132

Dr. Paul Scherer 6, 106, 107, 123

Dr. Steve Subotnick 17, 125

Dr. Ronald Valmassy 3, 25, 36, 125

Dr. John Weed 3, 76, 132

Dr. Justin Wernick 3

E

Early Heel Off 75-76

Elaine Root 18

Equinus Problems 31, 75-77

Everted Forefoot Deformities 106

Examples of Gait Findings with Treatment Options 81-84

Excessive Internal Patellar Rotation 79-80

Extensor Digitorum Longus Tendon Strength 114

Extensor Hallucis Longus Tendon Strength 113

F

Fall Program 102

Feehery Modification 19, 29, 50, 112, 121, 122

Feel of the Foot at Push-off 35-36

Femoral Stress Fractures 62

Fettig Technique 5, 19, 29, 112

Fifth Metatarsal Stress Fracture 59

Fibular Stress Fractures 61

Finding Subtalar Joint Neutral 110

First MPJ Pain 52

First Ray Cutout 99

First Ray Range of Motion 108-109

Flatness of Heel 46

Follow Up Advice in Injury Rehabilitation 43-44

Force Length Curve of Tendons 104

Forefoot Extensions 20

Forefoot Deformities 105-108

Forefoot Supinatus 23, 106

Forefoot Varus 23, 106, 125

Fourth Metatarsal Stress Fracture 59
Frontal Plane Abnormalities 32
Functional Hallux Limitus 52, 98-100
Functional Orthotic Devices for 2 Degrees Inversion 28

G

Gait Evaluation 9-11, 68-84
Gait Signs of Equinus 75-77
Gait Signs Over Pronation 70-71
Gait Signs Over Supination 71-74
Gait Signs Poor Shock Absorption 74-75
Gait Signs Short Leg Syndrome 69-70
Gait Signs Weak Muscles 77-81
Genu Recurvatum 75, 76-77
Genu Valgum 23, 25
Grading Orthotic Corrections 36
Growing Child and the Inverted Orthotic Technique 40-41

H

Haglund's Deformity 60
Hammertoes 52, 58
Hamstrings 55, 61
Hannaford Orthotic Device 123
Heel Motion in Gait 10-11
Heel Bisection 8,10, 12, 95-96
Heel Cups 19
Heel Lift 75-76, 79
Heel Position Change 3
Heel Valgus 23, 95
Highest Inversion Initially Ordered 29
Highest Inversion Ordered 128
High Pitched Subtalar Joint Axis 112
Hip Arthralgias 62

History of Injury 65
Home Exercise Program 32
How Much Correction Is Needed 27-28
Hubscher's Maneuver 99-100

I

Iliotibial Band 34, 55, 62
Impression Cast to follow changes in Forefoot Supinatus 127
Impression Cast Importance 18, 130-132
Improving Pronation Control Temporarily 38
Indications for Inverted Orthotic Technique 23-27
Influences on Heel Position 9
Initial Pronation Treatment 32
Initial Treatment Focus 31
Intrinsic Muscle Strain 52-53
Inverted Forefoot Deformities 106
Inverted Orthotic Standard Components 7, 49-50

J

Jack's Test 99-100
Jeffrey Root 18, 132
J Strap for Pronation Control 116
Juvenile Acquired Flat Feet 23, 25-26
Juvenile Bunion Deformities 23, 26-27

K

Kathy Root 18
Kirby Skives
    Lateral 112, 121, 122, 124
    Medial 21, 26, 37, 40, 111, 112, 124, 125, 126, 127
    Temporary 21-22, 122

Kinetic Wedge 16, 99
KLM Labs 125
Knee 54-55, 61

L

Langer Labs 16, 99
Late Midstance Pronation 77
Lateral Ankle Instability 58-60, 125
LCC or Lateral Column Correction 19, 122, 124
Lateral Column Support 5-6, 18, 29, 49-50
Lateral Kirby Skive 19, 34-35
Lateral Knee Collateral Ligament Sprain 61
Lateral Meniscus 17, 23, 25, 54
LEO correction 124
Lifts for Short Leg Syndrome 31, 94
Limb Length Discrepancy Landmarks 93-94
Low Back Pain 62-63
Low Dye Taping 116
Lowering Correction Techniques 7, 13, 34-35

M

Manipulation of Forefoot Supinatus Before Impression Casting 46
Manufacturing the Inverted Orthotic Technique 45-48
MCC or Medial Column Correction 21, 123-124, 125, 126, 127
Medial and Lateral Instability 124, 125
Medial Arch Height 18-19
Medial Column Enhancements Inverted Orthotic Technique 21-22
Medial Knee Pain from Over Supination 34, 61
Medial Shin Splints 17, 23, 25, 27
Metatarsalgia 52, 58-59

Metatarsal Roll at Push Off 34
Midsole Shoe Wedging 127
Midtarsal Joint Change in Motion with Pronation/Supination 16
Midtarsal Joint Range of Motion 112-113
MMS or Maximal Metatarsal Support 123
Mobilization for Tight Muscles 120
Mobilization of Forefoot Supinatus 106
Modification if the Foot doesn't Clear the Arch 128-129
Modifications for Over Supination 34-35
Modified Root Device 23, 123, 125, 127
Morton's Neuroma/Neuritis 52

N

Neutral Calcaneal Stance Position 97
Neutral Tibial Position 97-98
Normal Physiological Length 104

O

Occam's Law 65, 67
Orthotic Therapy as a Process 24
Orthotic Functions 1, 58
Orthotic Type based on Function 30
Outsole Varus Wedging 83
Out Toe Gait 77
Over Correction 38, 58
Over Pronation Initial Treatment 32
Over Pronation Gait Findings 70-71
Over Pronation Symptoms 56-57
Over Supination Gait Findings 71-74
Over Supination Symptoms 58-64
Over The Counter Inserts 4, 32-33, 115

P

Pain Level for Healing 43

Pain Produced by Over Pronation 52-57

Pain Produced by Over Supination 58-64

Partially Compensated Rearfoot Varus 111-112

Patellofemoral Injuries 17, 23, 25, 54

Patient Involvement in the Inverted Orthotic Technique Process 30

Peroneal Strain from Over Supination 34, 60

Peroneus Brevis Tendon Strength 113

Peroneus Longus Tendon 16, 53, 60

Peroneus Longus Tendon Strength 113

Peroneus Tertius Tendon Strength 113

Pes Anserinus Tendonitis/Bursitis 54

Pes Cavus 124, 126

Phalanges (orthotic) 19

Phases of Rehabilitation 41, 67

Piriformis Syndrome 17, 55

Plan B use of the Inverted Orthotic Technique 28, 65

Planes of Deformity 24, 89-91

Plantar Fasciitis 53

Positive Casts 46

Posterior Tibial Tendon 16, 53

Posterior Tibial Tendon Dysfunction 23, 25, 36, 82-84, 101, 127

Posterior Tibial Tendon Strength 113

Posterior Tibial Tendon Taping 83, 116

Poor Heel Lift 79

Power Lacing 24, 68, 127

Powerstep Inserts 32, 115

Process of the Inverted Orthotic Technique 30

ProLab USA 107, 123

Prolonged Heat Ice Stretch 120

Pronation Categories 24

Pronation Initial Treatment 32

Pronation Support Modalities 2, 43, 115-117

Proximal Tib-Fib Sprain 61

Push Off Sense 35-36

R

Raising Lateral Support Adjustments 13

Raising Medial Support Adjustments 13

Rearfoot Varus and Inverted Orthotic Technique 17, 20

Rehabilitation General Rules 41, 43

References for the Inverted Orthotic Technique 136-137

Relaxed Calcaneal Stance Position 26, 29, 94

Relaxed Calcaneal Stance Position with Heel Valgus 23

Robert Blake 131

Rocker Bottom Flat Foot 75

Role of Weak and Tight Muscles 118-121

Root Functional Orthotic Device 23, 122-123, 124

Root Functional Orthotic Laboratory 18, 25, 132

Rule of 3 for Injuries 31, 65, 81, 82

Running Landing Position 14, 24

Running Less Stress Produced By 15

Running Limb Varus 125, 126

Running Orthotic Devices 15, 24, 125, 127-128

Running Store Rule on Pes Cavus 73-74

Runners Utilizing Inverted Technique 14

Runner's Wedges 17, 18, 115

S

Sacroiliac Symptoms from Over Supination 34, 62

Sagittal Plane Blockade 16, 99

Sagittal Plane Deformities 24, 32

Sagittal Plane Pronation 23, 24

Sciatic Nerve 25

Second Metatarsal Stress Fracture 52

Second MPJ Pain 52

Separate Running and Walking Orthotic Devices 126
Serial Orthotic Devices with the Inverted Orthotic Technique 39-40
Sesamoid Pain 52
Shin Splints 17, 23, 27
Shock Absorption 74-75
Shoes for Supinators 74
Shoe Influence on Correction 15
Shoe Influence on Over Supination 64
Shoe Variations for Rehabilitation 42
Short Leg Syndrome 69-70
Side Lean 80
Single Heel Raise Evaluation 101
Single Leg Balancing 102
Sinus Tarsi Syndrome 53
Soft Based Orthotic Devices 123
Sole Inserts 32, 115
Soleus Strain 53
Squinting Patella 79-80
Stability Components towards Better Health 45
Stabilizing Orthotic Device 122-123
Staging Orthotic Correction 36-37
Standing Heel Position 8
Starting Point Inverted Orthotic Device 4
Steppage Gait 79
Strengthening for Pronation Control 43, 116, 119
Strengthening for Supination Control 119
Strengthening General Rules 114, 119
Strengthening Types of Exercises 114
Stretching for Pronation Control 116
Stretching for Excessively Tight Tendons 120
Stretching Principles 118-119
Subtalar Joint Axis 112
Subtalar Joint Neutral Position 109-112
Support the Foot Taping 116
"S" Word 83

T

Tailor's Bunions 59
Tarsal Tunnel Syndrome 23, 25, 39-40, 53, 111-112
Taping 32, 83, 116
Temple University Stretch 120
Tentative Diagnosis 65
Tibial Stress Fractures 53
Tibial Varum 18, 97-98, 111, 125, 126
Transverse Plane Deformities 25, 32
Transverse Plane Pronation 23, 24-25
Trendelenburg Gait 80
Tri-axial Orthosis 4

U

UCBL 7
Under Correction Reasons 38-39

V

Valgus Wedges 20, 32
Valgus Midsole Wedge 20
Varying Stresses as Healthy Part of Rehabilitation 42
Varus Midsole Wedge 14, 21, 127
Varus Outsole Wedge 21
Varus Wedges 18, 21, 115
Video Anti-Supination Modifications 20
Video Impression Casting 132
Video Inverted Technique 1
Visit (Goal of first visit) 4

W

Weakest Link in the Chain 84

Weak Muscles causing Pronation 32
Weight Bearing Stress in Inverted Orthotic
Device 16

X

X-ray for Short Leg 70

Y

YouTube Channel 3

Inverted Orthotic Technique Answers to Pre-Test

1. What is the number one function of the Inverted Orthotic Technique? The Inverted Orthotic Technique places a varus force in the rearfoot to change pronation stresses

2. If a patient stands 12 degrees everted in heel valgus, what is the initial Inverted Orthotic Technique degrees ordered? 35 degrees

3. How does the cast correction correlate to the degrees of heel change noted for the patient? 5 degrees of cast correction correlates to 1 degree of heel inversion

4. What are the common muscle groups strengthened in patients who have pronation syndrome? Intrinsic foot muscles, posterior and anterior tibial, peroneus longus, gastrocnemius and soleus, lateral hamstrings, pes anserinus, external hip rotators

5. With a resting position of 2 degrees inverted, how can that be related to a pronation problem? When there is a high degree of tibial varum, the patient pronate excessively and still not get the heel to a vertical position. This is called a partially compensated rearfoot varus condition.

6. With overpronation, which knee compartment gets compressed? Lateral compartment gets compressed, so controlling pronation can help lateral meniscal problems especially if some varus force can be generated to open up the lateral joint line.

7. As you attempt to eliminate or slow down overpronation, what are methods utilized to protect the lateral column from oversupination? High lateral heel cups, lateral phalanges to the orthotic device, forefoot extensions with more support under the 4th and 5th metatarsal heads, Denton modifications, lateral flare or extension distally to the normal rearfoot post, maximal midtarsal joint pronation in the suspension cast, Feehery or Fettig modifications to the Inverted Orthotic Technique, lateral column corrections and lateral Kirbys, and less medial force with narrower orthotic device, lower medial heel cup, removal of the medial ½ rearfoot post or some of the medial aspect, plantar fascial groove, thinning medial arch, and utilizing less rigid plastic material.

8. Why does equinus cause excessive pronation, in what plane primarily does it cause subluxation, and why is it important to reverse when utilizing the Inverted Orthotic Technique? Equinus forces can produce a sagittal plane subluxation arch collapse just following middle of midstance as the body weight moves over the midfoot. The Inverted Orthotic Technique produces a high arch which will fight the equinus force trying to collapse the arch. The equinus force may win causing arch pain from the war being waged, or an early heel lift may occur, or the hip make compensate

with excessive angle of gait, or the knee may be forced into genu recurvatum damaging the knee. Best strategy is to recognize the equinus soon, and begin to stretch out the tightness.

9. When designing an Inverted Orthotic Device, what landmark becomes the peak of the medial arch? Navicular 1st Cuneiform Joint

10. When performing gait evaluations, what are the 6 most common abnormal forces you are evaluating for that you can begin to treat? Excessive pronation, excessive supination, limb length difference, poor shock absorption, tight muscles and weak muscles

11. There are 27 common areas that can get painful from overpronation listed (Appendix 1). What are the 3 most common sources of pain in the distal medial shin from overpronation? Posterior Tibial Muscle/Tendon, Soleus Muscle, Tibial Periosteum or bone itself

12. Overpronation, if it is the cause or aggravating factor in an injury, affects the weakest link in the chain. If it affects a weak posterior tibial tendon, what are the 7 locations that a weak posterior tibial tendon can present with pain? Tibial attachment with stress fracture, periosteum, muscle belly, tendon, navicular attachment, os tibial externum, and plantar arch with distal fibres

13. From simple to complex, what are the 10 methods of helping to control overpronation (for example, one of

them is J strap heel inversion with leukotape and coverall to protect the skin)? Stable shoes, power lacing, OTC arch supports, varus wedges as shoe insert, arch taping like Low Dye or Quick Tape from supportthefoot.com, , muscle strengthening, tendon stretching with equinus, customizing OTC arch supports, J Strap for slight heel inversion, custom foot orthotic devices

14. The Inverted Orthotic Technique is made off of what 2 casting techniques at present? Suspension Casting and Digital Scanners both performed with subtalar joint neutral and midtarsal joints maximally pronated

15. Why does one patient with overpronation get well with 25% pronation help and another patient needs 110% for awhile? At times the correction needs to only take the joints out of their subluxation range back into a normal range of motion, and at other times, the position of the foot has to be a certain temporarily or permanently to prevent further breakdown (example of preventing early Stage III PTTD from progressing into Stage IV and the need for surgery).

16. Occam's Law means that the most common cause of an injury is the cause of the injury. How does this work with the Rule of 3 in the investigation of the cause of many overuse injuries? The example I use often is regarding tibial sesamoid

injuries. The common overuse case of tibial sesamoid injuries is overpronation which nobody denies. The Rule of 3 forces you to look for other causes that can help in the treatment including actual bone health (Vit D deficiency or low bone density), the individual foot biomechanics like plantarflexed first ray, the type of shoe worn like minimalist without good plantar foot protection, or training habits of poor recovery times and too much sidewalk running).